'This book should be given to every female in Western society as soon as they can read' *Anon*, UK

'*Women's Pleasure* contain the author devised for hersel ich was rich, full and happy b ed in a style which is blissf d, **SUNDAY EXPRESS**

'A remarkable and unequivocal study of female sexuality' MAIL ON SUNDAY

'Witty, sensible and forthright . . . she doesn't pussyfoot around, is never coy and assumes that all women deserve, and can achieve, the big O, over and over' LUDUS MAGAZINE

'Thank you for writing such a brilliant book. I've only just started the programme but I already feel so much happier in myself . . . What scares me is that I might never have read the article in the *Mail on Sunday* about your book. The thought of not reading your book and getting what I want from sex, well . . .' *Ms J. M.*, Devon

'This is one book I desperately need. Sod the Penguin Classics' *Anon*, (London)

'Oh yes! Oh yes! Oh yes!' MRS A. B., (Aylesbury)

'Her central theme of regaining control over one's sexuality goes to the core of why some women can't climax . . . A lot of clean fun' WEEKLY JOURNAL

'I have immense amounts I could tell you, but I'll write again when I've finished the book. I'd just like to say, thank God you finally wrote it' C., (Watford) (age 29)

'Well written, well researched . . . riveting' SUNDAY INDEPENDENT (Ireland)

'As amusing as it is helpful . . . a wonderful understanding of the baggage women bring to bed' NEW WOMAN (Australia)

'A courageous, witty and controversial book' MORE MAGAZINE (New Zealand)

'I have also read a few books on sex, but have found them very clinical or plain rubbish . . . At last somebody has the nerve to put into words what most women would dare not say, "Help, I need an orgasm" ' MS M. T., (Manchester)

'This has to be one of the best books I have read for a long time. Thank you so much for your refreshing and realistic look at women's potential to orgasm. I am in half a mind to lend this to my boyfriend to read tonight. Most of all, it has inspired me to confront the issue and my boyfriend and to work on being honest about what I really desire. Thank you again!' MS L.A., (London)

'. . . enjoyable and thought provoking. My husband and I have both read it through and have been discussing it madly. I wanted to thank you for your book and more importantly for writing and speaking so candidly about the subject . . .' MRS V.H., (N.Z.)

'I enjoyed your book and will pass it on to my sister eventually. I especially like the chapter on oral sex where you give some scenarios – Number 5 was a classic – it's happened several times to me and when I read it in print, I broke up with laughter. I thought I was the only one with that problem.' MS L. D., (Perth)

'I think that it will not only help myself but also help me to deliver a more exciting Health Education Course to my eleventh-year students' MS G, (North Humberside)

'Congratulations on your wonderful book, which was long overdue. It will certainly give much needed information and reassurance to many women and much needed information to many men' MS L. C., (South Africa) (age 37)

'Your ideas are wonderful especially for 'Islamic Society' . . . I hope I get the opportunity to smuggle your book to these countries in their own language' DR A., (Edinburgh)

WOMEN'S PLEASURE

or

*How to have an Orgasm
as often as you want*

RACHEL SWIFT

PAN BOOKS

First published 1993 by Pan Books

This edition published 1994 by Pan Books
an imprint of Macmillan Publishers Ltd
25 Eccleston Place, London SW1W 9NF
Basingstoke and Oxford
Associated companies throughout the world
www.macmillan.co.uk

ISBN 0 330 33325 9

9 8

A CIP catalogue record for this book is available from
the British Library.

Typeset by Cambridge Composing (UK) Ltd, Cambridge
Printed and bound in Great Britain by
Mackays of Chatham PLC, Chatham, Kent

CONTENTS

PART ONE

PART TWO

PART THREE

DEDICATION

This new edition of *Women's Pleasure* is dedicated to the many women and men (from all over the world) who have written to me in support of the book. Although the sheer number of letters has made it impossible for me to reply to them individually, I have read every one with grateful appreciation.

The author and publishers wish to thank the following who have kindly given permission for the use of copyright materials.

Virgin Publishing Ltd for extracts from Appolinaire's *The Exploits of a Young Don Juan*;
Hello! Limited for extracts from an interview with Angelica Houston by Anna Maria Bahann;
Little, Brown for extracts from *The Hite Report on Male Sexuality*.

Every effort has been made to trace all the copyright holders but if any has been inadvertently overlooked, the author and publishers will be pleased to make the necessary arrangement at the first opportunity.

PART ONE

CHAPTER ONE

WHAT EXACTLY IS THIS BOOK?

This is a selfish book.

I am an average woman in her thirties who until recently had never once had an orgasm during sex with her partner. There was nothing wrong with me. I didn't hate sex or find my partners distasteful. I didn't have insurmountable psychological difficulties about men, penises, or letting myself go. I was, physically and emotionally, an ordinary woman. Yet the simple and pleasant experience of orgasm during sex seemed beyond my reach.

One day, after a particularly frustrating encounter, I decided I was sick and tired of it. I'd had my fill of going to bed with men who would climax without any trouble at all, while I was left with no recourse but to tip-toe to the bathroom and finish myself off in secret. So I determined to *teach* myself to have an orgasm *whenever I wanted one*.

This book explains how I did it. It is a straightforward, easy-to-follow, self-help plan that can teach you how to have as many orgasms as you want, whenever you want, with or without the full co-operation of your partner.

Who should read this book? Every woman in the world – and every woman's man. If you have never had an orgasm, this book will teach you how to do so. If you have them sometimes, it will show you that 'sometimes' can be doubled. If you're celibate, then you'll find plenty of fascinating facts and anecdotes to entertain you before you go to sleep. And if you're a man, it will teach you a

3

thing or two about how to be the sort of man a woman wants in her bed.

This book is also my story. Above all it is a positive story: sometimes funny, sometimes shocking. It is not written by an impersonal doctor or a soft-spoken therapist, but by a fellow malcontent who faced a difficult problem and found out for herself how to overcome it. It is, in other words, a book that deals with *realities* not ideals – what sex is really like, not what it is supposed to be like according to the manuals.

WHAT IS AN ORGASM?

Some people regard orgasm as the most intense feeling of physical pleasure there is. In describing it they become quite poetic: 'poised, pulsating – glowing', 'floating', 'an ecstatic frenzy of love, energy and emotion, all mixed together', 'supreme sensitivity to touch – waves of butterflies in my stomach', 'hot', 'beautiful and *alive*', 'open and languorous', 'electric currents blowing through my body', 'voluptuous, elegant and sensuous', 'my whole body burns', 'an experience that is somehow spiritual as well as physical', and of course 'eager for more'.

The word itself derives from the Greek *orgao* (swell). The *Oxford English Dictionary* defines it as a 'paroxysm of desire or rage or other passion'. Without going into technical language it is perhaps best described as a few brief moments leading up to the highest peak of sexual desire, followed by a pleasurable, perhaps over-whelming, sense of release. Orgasms are concentrated on the genitals but, as the descriptions above make clear, radiate to all parts of the body. Many people experience a corresponding wave of emotion.

It is also true that orgasms – particularly female ones – vary greatly in intensity. Occasionally they are mild, even disappointing sensations. Some women are uncertain whether they've experi-enced one or not, though this is unusual.

There is, however, another answer to the question 'What is an orgasm?' For many women it is a battlefield. Often the man's orgasm is considered a necessary consequent of good sex, while hers is just a happy extra – good news if she gets it done in time, but not to be fretted over if she's a little too slow, or too tense, or the sex hasn't been good enough. Because it may be difficult for her to climax, orgasm can become an unforgettable issue – not helped by the implicit suggestion that today unless a woman has a whopping great climax on time, in time, and with loads of groans and gasps into the bargain, she has somehow not managed to come up to scratch.

WHY ALL THIS CONCENTRATION ON ORGASM?

A close friend of mine, who knew I was writing this book, asked a pertinent question. 'Is it really such a good idea to write a book that concentrates solely on orgasm? After all, orgasm is only one element of sex – there's so much more to a relationship than orgasm.'

I agree with her wholeheartedly. I would never undervalue love, affection, commitment and understanding. They are essential ingredients of a successful relationship, and very helpful for good sex too. But it is not my place to talk about such matters – everyone will conduct their relationships in their own special ways and I'm not about to interfere. Orgasm, on the other hand, *is* something I can help with. I know from personal experience the kind of problems women suffer, and I know from personal experience how to help them.

'But,' continued my friend, 'is orgasm really that valuable? After all, many women lead happy and fulfilling lives without it.'

This is an attitude I came across often during my own training and research, and I think it misses the point. I believe that for sexually active women orgasm *is* an issue, at some level. At the very least it's not something we can ever forget about, as one fellow sufferer made clear: 'I see *him* do it, day after day, *of course* it means something to me. I want to be able to share that.' Another

5

commented, 'You'd have to be deaf, dumb and blind not to think about orgasm. I mean, nowadays sex is just *everywhere*. Why should we, as women, take second best, when our potential is so great?'

Shere Hite, who questioned 3500 women between the ages of fourteen and seventy-eight, quotes case after case of women who felt 'depressed', 'tense', 'cheated and envious', 'less desirable', 'incomplete', 'frustrated', 'insecure' – and so on. Hite unhesitatingly concludes: 'Almost every woman who didn't orgasm would like to.' In a society where orgasm *is* an issue, constantly reinforced by films, books and endless unsatisfactory sexual encounters, it would be arrogant of me to pretend I could upset the *status quo* by claiming that women ought not to take orgasm so seriously. What I *can* do is show that difficulty with orgasm is not so serious. If you want, you can do something about it.

Although I do not maintain that orgasm is a necessity for good sex, I firmly believe that for women it is important as an *option*. To make an analogy: when education was denied women, it was commonly believed that they were all empty-headed dimwits. Only when education became available could women prove that they were the intellectual equals of men. It is a similar story with orgasm: the myth of male sexual superiority is alive and well, yet the truth is that most women have simply not had the *opportunity* to fulfil their very great sexual potential.

You, as an individual, may choose not to enrol in higher education, just as you may choose not to insist on orgasm every time you have sex. But we all need to have access to orgasm before we can decide whether it is for us or not. Once we have learned all about it, *then* we can decide how important it is in our lives.

WHAT ABOUT MY PARTNER?

Although I have called this a 'selfish' book, it has a very unselfish result. A satisfying sex life helps relationships as well as individuals. The more a woman is able to enjoy sex fully with her partner, the more the partner and the relationship will benefit. And I don't just mean in the bedroom, but in all sorts of non-sexual ways, because sexual dissatisfaction is, famously, the cause of a great deal of emotional and social tension outside the bedroom.

This book is as valuable for those who have been married thirty-five years as for those who change their partner once a week. However, it is a fundamental principle of the plan that women help themselves. For this reason the exercises do *not* require a permanent or willing and compliant partner. Let's face it, not everybody has such a person. In fact much of the programme – particularly the crucial early steps – must be done by a woman on her own. The later steps can be done without the man being aware that you are following a training programme. I have suggested techniques to get your man to co-operate unknowingly. The end result, *for both of you*, will be well worth a little guile.

Those of you who have a patient and caring partner have the choice whether or not to involve him in your training programme. But think about it carefully. The fact of a person of the opposite sex being concerned in such a sensitive, intimate matter may be unsettling. When he is there with you, doing everything exactly as he should, you may feel guilty and unwilling to disappoint him. He may be the ideal man, but if he shares in the knowledge that you are trying to achieve orgasm, the sense of public expectation can make you awkward, as if performing on stage. The very closeness of the relationship can, paradoxically, inhibit you. Besides, even if you do have such a partner, you may have been faking some or all of your orgasms up till now, and it would require some pretty delicate talking to get round that! If, however, you feel that your partner's knowledge and assistance in the plan will help you, bring him into your confidence.

Best of all: follow the programme on your own for the first three or four steps. Then decide whether you tell your partner. Perhaps, once you have seen the great strides you are making, you will feel it important to discuss the matter. Perhaps you will prefer to keep it your secret for always. That is your choice.

HOW DO I USE THIS BOOK?

Many women – and, I hope, men – will be content simply to read this book through, like any other. There's plenty of interest in it for everybody.

Those of you who also wish to follow the self-help plan should take account of the following.

Whatever your starting point, my method aims to build up your confidence and introduce you gradually to techniques, so that you advance in sensible stages. Each step represents a significant success; at the end of each one I recommend that you *celebrate*. You'll then be in an excellent frame of mind to go on to the next stage.

As I was devising the plan, step by step, I passed on my tips and discoveries to friends and acquaintances. These 'guinea pigs', who ranged in age from seventeen to sixty-one and were of very different social backgrounds, reported extremely successful results. During the course of this book they will be speaking for themselves.

I have also made free use of Shere Hite's two great tomes, *The Hite Report on Female Sexuality* and *The Hite Report on Male Sexuality*. This is because there are occasions when I wish to make it clear that a particular point is not simply a crazy idea of mine, but an opinion endorsed by thousands. Hite's researches were extremely broad-ranging: she questioned not only 3500 women as mentioned above, but also over 7000 men from thirteen to seventy-nine. Her books do not suffer from the sense of impersonality and scientific callousness that pervades many such studies. Her questions and comments are intelligent and wide-ranging, but not ridiculously cautious. They are without obvious bias. Hite allows the respondents to reply at length, and does not ask them to give merely a yes or no. And, of course, Hite is a woman.

*

This book contains eighteen chapters.

Part One: Chapters 1 to 4 are introductory. It is important that you read these so as to appreciate the function and motivation behind the plan and the style in which it is presented.

Part Two: Chapter 5 is a preparation for the plan. Among other things this includes a very personal questionnaire about some of the issues covered by the book. Chapters 6 to 13 comprise the plan itself: six main steps and two side-steps. If steps and side-steps sound complicated, let me assure you that, on the contrary, they are arranged like this for the greatest possible flexibility to sui: your own needs. Read through these chapters carefully before you begin to get a picture of how the plan works, and to see if you need to make any adjustments in your sexual relationship with your partner in preparation for the later steps which involve his presence.

You must progress through each of the main steps carefully and in sequence. As with learning a language, each step must be practised to the full, so keep on one until you are thoroughly comfortable with it. Your patience will be rewarded in the end.

Once you have perfected a step, move on to the next. *But don't stop practising the previous step*. Throughout this programme you should be consolidating your gains even while you're learning new skills.

The side-steps can be introduced at any time after step 2. It depends on when you feel comfortable about them.

Part Three: the remaining chapters are on a variety of issues relating to women's orgasms. Read whichever you feel might be important to you, before you begin the programme. Chapter 18 has been written especially for men.

Always bear in mind the really good news: the ability to have an orgasm, *whenever* you want one, achieved through careful training and practice, is yours to keep. Like riding a bike. You will need to keep up your expertise by repeating old exercises now and then. Occasionally circumstances will be against you – a really selfish lump of a partner, for example, or too many glasses of wine! But once you have really mastered the art of orgasm you will not readily lose that ability. The achievement *is yours for life*.

CHAPTER TWO

MY STORY

Madame shall we undress you for the fight?
The wars are naked that we make tonight.

(G. Moore, *Memoirs of My Dead Life*)

There used to be a rather unpleasant girl at my school called
Sophy. She had 'advanced' parents and was president of the Love
Club. The members of the club had to rack their parents' bookshelves for any mention of 'love', then meet the next day behind a
tree in the playground and gloat over the most enticing bits.

'*He gripped her passionately*,' read Lorna one day in a thrilling
voice, from a messy-looking paperback stolen from her father's
study. '*His hands slid slowly down her throat, and she could feel his
throbbing lips—*'

'Ugh!'

'Shut *up*!'

'Well, it says so here, look – "*throbbing*".'

'I feel sick.'

At this sophisticated juncture the Love Club meetings would
usually degenerate into fights and giggles. But this time Sophy
only smiled knowingly. 'I'll bet you half a bag of toffees you don't
know what an "orgasm" is.'

'If it's anything to do with throbbing I'm going home.'

'How do you spell it?' I asked, trying to keep the minutes up to
date.

Lorna haggled over the price. Eventually the bargain was struck,
and Sophy lowered her voice.

'*It's when your father goes to the loo inside your mother!*'

We burst into uproar.

At a later meeting Sophy – who was an authority on everything outré – announced that she knew what men and women *really* did with each other in private.

'Well?' We all crowded round.

'They go upside-down on the bed and lick each other.'

'*What?*' we cried in chorus, horrified.

'I *know*,' said Sophy. 'I *saw*.'

When we had recovered from this bombshell, Petra leaned forward:

'Once you let a man have his way with you, he'll leave you in the lurch,' she announced confidently.

'What's the lurch?' asked Fanny.

'My mother says never make the first move with a man or you'll scare him off,' somebody else added.

'Men are different from women,' said Sophy. 'They have to sleep with plenty of girls before they marry because it's "in their nature". Otherwise, if they bottle it up it all explodes later.'

'*Explodes?*'

'Yes, and they run away with someone else.'

I remember looking at my little brother and thinking that surely there must be exceptions. Yet it was he who brought the matter up next.

'What is sex?' he asked plaintively at breakfast one morning. Our parents looked appalled – he was only seven.

'Why do you ask a thing like that?' mumbled my mother.

'Because I want to send off for a cowboy outfit and it says "state sex".'

Sex – and particularly orgasm – was a strange, somewhat distasteful subject. My parents used to talk now and then of the male and female sex, but these were subjects quite far removed from the sex that Sophy knew so much about. The female sex, for example, had 'duties'.

'However much of a high-flier you become, a man likes to be looked after,' reminded my father. 'After all, it's a woman's duty to make the home.'

'We made bullets during the war,' muttered my mother.

'This is peace,' my father replied firmly.

I had a violent crush on Terry Thomas, and couldn't help feeling that the dim-witted dolly birds with their wiggling hips, high heels and empty eyes were far beneath him. I particularly admired the way he used to leap out of an open sports car and adjust his tie.

'An awful smoothie,' said my father. 'Nice girls wouldn't be taken in. I can tell you that much for a fact,' he continued, unconsciously adjusting his own tie.

'Oh, be quiet, Peter,' said my mother.

But even she, whom I now realize was in many ways a remarkable woman ahead of her time, agreed that it was death to be ambitious with men. 'Every man wants to marry a pure woman,' she warned darkly, when at seventeen I was flying out of the house to a party. I was horrified when I overheard an unmarried male friend confide to my father, 'What I always say is, if you want a girl for the night, go for the plain ones. They're so grateful for the attention, they'll do anything you ask.'

PROGRESS?

Along came the Swinging Sixties and I let my hair down and my mini skirts crept higher and higher. I remember my first pair of embroidered bell-bottoms – I also remember my parents' expression when I waltzed into their dinner party wearing them. Now I could walk through the neighbourhood with a man twice running without Mrs Wigglesworth leaning over the fence to ask my father if I intended 'to make a commitment to him'.

I brought back boyfriends, then took them away again and had a bit of a feel around in the back of their car or at a party, before the ordeal of remounting the creaking stairs at three in the morning. 'We'll always love you, you know,' said my parents, thinking that the whole decade was little more than an extended adolescent rebellion. They tried to take in these developments, although my father couldn't help making his little jokes about the 'new *dis*order'.

Sophy's images of sex still haunted me, especially the thought of being used as a *pissoir* by my future husband, but I kept these strange ideas at the back of my mind. One day a boy I'd met in a coffee shop took me to a film and afterwards we ended up in his 'den' at the bottom of his parents' garden. Then he lay on top of me, pressing his penis down on my stomach and squirming about. Pretty quickly he seemed to lose control, which had never happened with my other boyfriends. I wondered if he was having a fit and if I should get him dressed again and call his parents. Suddenly it was all over.

'Did you "explode"?' I asked.

Then I went away to university in another town. One day a student from the geography department whom I had taken a fancy to sat down at my table. He was tall and chunky with a slight swagger about him that impressed me for its independence. He wore dark glasses and had a sort of contemptuous smile that wasn't really directed at anything in particular. I thought this immensely cool. At a party that weekend he gave me something to smoke which made me cough and splutter. Then he gave me a drink which nearly knocked me flat. I remember dancing and a taxi ride to a far-flung corner of the city. I remember undressing, and the smell of joss sticks, the sound of Mick Jagger singing 'Satisfaction'. I remember that we both passed out, but I don't remember whether it was that night that I lost my virginity or the following morning.

When I went to visit him again he was playing music very loud and had dimmed all the lights. He got rid of the friend he was talking to by explaining, with an ill-concealed wink, that he had some business to attend to, and then he took off my clothes slowly, holding a glass in one hand, touching every part of me and commenting as he did so. 'It was fabulous last night, wasn't it?' he muttered in my ear, as he pulled off his underpants. 'You enjoyed it, didn't you?' I said yes, and felt a little foolish that I couldn't remember anything about it. 'I could tell that you did, I could *tell*,' he murmured. Then he pulled me on to the carpet, and as he entered me he whispered, 'I'll make you come.'

To be fair, Gerry was just a puffed-up young man who'd been thrown in at the deep end by a decade that had more daring than understanding; he probably matured in time and became a nice, sensitive individual. But it still annoys the hell out of me that it never occurred to him that sex was anything more than a display of his penile prowess. My climax was, in his eyes, a test which either he could pass or I could fail. And by making me afraid of failure he pretty well ensured it. All Gerry saw was that he had performed a heroic deed. Therefore when I didn't groan and wail at the appropriate moment, there must have been something wrong with *me*.

The next couple of years saw a string of casual boyfriends: after all, in those days it was just assumed that you'd sleep together right away. Sometimes it was nice, sometimes bloody awful, mostly neither. One day I met a man in the library whom I liked a lot. He was elegant, not too studious, and he seemed particularly keen on me, which is always a bonus. We went out to supper a few times, then back to my flat where we made love for about half an hour in front of a new electric fire I'd just bought and was very proud of.

'Did you come?' he asked breathlessly when he'd finished.

'No, but it doesn't matter, I enjoyed it a lot.'

'Have you ever come?' he asked, after a pause.

'No.'

'Haven't you had an orgasm *ever*?' he asked again, quietly. 'Not with *any* man?'

'No,' I admitted, beginning to think that he seemed quite concerned.

'Oh.' His face lit up with relief. 'Then it's hardly my fault, is it?'

Sometimes I didn't tell, but just hoped for the best. Quite often a man would simply ignore whether I had or hadn't come – in those days women's orgasms were not the hot news they are now. But of course if you didn't 'confess' beforehand there was always the risk that right in the midst of a passionate moment your lover would mutter, 'Haven't you *come* yet? We've been doing it for twenty minutes, you know.'

Why didn't I fake an orgasm? Quite simply it never occurred to me. And by the time I was tipped off about this by another woman, I didn't have the confidence. To begin with I was not sure *how* you faked one. Secondly I was quite convinced that a man would be able to spot it at once. After all, men were the ones who had all the experience, weren't they?

Naturally, not all men were like this. The bad ones stick out in my memory simply because they played heavily upon my sexual sensitivity. My first husband, on the other hand, was a wonderful man: kind, considerate and a real expert in bed. He made me feel better between the sheets than I'd ever felt before and introduced me to sex that seemed almost indecently hot. Thinking about it even now gives me a tingling feeling – I hate to think how many times we got close to being caught at parties and official functions. And I enjoyed the sex. Often I enjoyed it so much that I reached a peak of agonized and unrelieved frustration, constantly (as it seemed) on the brink of relief but never getting there. I could have screamed. But I never had an orgasm.

Nowadays I sometimes *choose* not to reach orgasm during sex – if I'm feeling lazy or particularly mellow. And that in itself is pleasurable because I know that I can come when I want to. But until recently I found it deeply frustrating to feel I was unable to climax, no matter what my desires.

MY FAULT, OR HIS?

The more I observed my partner lying in blissful contentment beside me, the more I was convinced that there was something wrong with me. Not something obvious that could be put right, but something secret, deep down, that was stopping me climax and that perhaps I could never ever cure. Films, books, magazines, articles, all testified to the fact that I was the odd one out. Other women climaxed happily without any difficulty. None of my friends gave any signs that they were ever dissatisfied with the way their bodies functioned during nights on the tiles. If I pressed for details – pretending, of course, that I just wanted to hear a titillating story – the happy woman either went coy or boastful, assuring me that she'd enjoyed it like there was no tomorrow.

I remember getting into intimate conversation with a special friend of mine, who seemed just the sort who might also have trouble – she'd been anorexic for a long time and was generally nervous and unconfident. She'd been having an affair with a man about twelve years older than herself.

'Well, tell me all,' I urged. 'Is he good in bed?'

'Oh, he's really decent,' she said quietly. 'He always waits for me to climax before doing so himself.'

One more blow.

Sometimes I wished I were truly 'frigid' – unable to feel anything at all – then at least, I felt, I could either give the whole thing up as a bad job and lead a pleasant life on my own, or find some really obvious difficulty I could grasp hold of.

It wasn't even as if I was a meek little thing who was accustomed to accepting second best. In other aspects of life I was pretty demanding. I could do just about everything that a man was traditionally supposed to be able to do, so why not this? I could fix a motor car, run a house, build cupboards. I was intelligent and resourceful. I could run faster than anyone in the office (I found that out when we had a charity sports day. I also won the egg and spoon race). I once even beat up a burglar – not with my handbag, but with a jab from my elbow and a kick at his kneecap. There wasn't anything obviously wrong with my childhood. I read of women who had suffered trauma, either physical or mental, and lost the satisfaction they had once been able to have, or had never gained. I even read of one poor newly-wed whose husband had dropped her when crossing the threshold and knocked out her orgasm as well as her! But I had none of those excuses. And the most maddening and inexplicable thing of all was that I could make myself come as many times as I liked when I was on my own.

Then, in the mid-eighties, came the fear of AIDS. Suddenly the *quality* of sex – not the quantity – became important as never before. Many of my friends felt that they had had enough of wild promiscuity; some had settled down. Though divorced from my first husband I myself had a flourishing career which took me to a lot of conferences – where in turn I met a lot of men. Soon I was again settled into a comfortable relationship. I had matured quite a bit, felt more at ease with myself in a variety of ways. I had learned something of the kind of lovemaking I enjoyed. *But still no orgasm.* However satisfactory, and however long my partner was able to continue, I knew that orgasm was a long way away. I was, I realized bleakly, one of those women who would never have an orgasm.

And I didn't like it one bit.

REVELATIONS

Then I began working among a group of women. After a pleasant partnership of several weeks, we went for a celebratory supper at an Indian restaurant. The wine flowed very freely and we began chatting. In the early hours of the following morning we had moved to someone's flat and were still chatting. Our subject? Sex. Tongues loosened by this time, the women talked about their husbands and lovers.

They talked about the size of their men's organs, of their fantasies, and of their sexual escapades – all the usual things. But unusually for me, who had always remained secretive about my sense of failure, they talked most of all *about their lack of sexual fulfilment*.

What was *doubly* astonishing to me was that they talked about sexual unfulfilment as if it were an obvious fact of life! They described unblushingly nights of frustration, of masturbation alone, and of faking orgasm – as if it were the most natural thing in the world.

It was a revelation. How naïve I had been! And those women were only the beginning of my understanding, because I was certain there was nothing very special about them. If they didn't enjoy sexual fulfilment, then the world must be full of women who didn't. I thought back to all those previous girlfriends of my partners, those enviable women who 'always had an orgasm', and I realized that of course they didn't '*always*'. Often as not they would have been faking or quite likely the men simply assumed they'd been satisfied without bothering to find out. I began to think of this problem in a brand new light.

After that, whenever I got the opportunity I deliberately steered the conversation with other friends on to sexual matters. Now I asked them what I wanted to know directly. Sure enough, among all the accounts of successful or remarkable sex – and there were quite a few of these – story after story poured out of disappointments, frustrations and distaste. Quite a number, like me, had never had an orgasm; many *were* able to orgasm, but only some of the time. 'It's a terribly hit-and-miss affair,' declared one woman. 'I just have to take pot luck.' A lot of them, like the women in the restaurant, were very funny about it – not in the least tragic, but treating it as a situation they had to accept. What did bother them was that they felt it was more than just a personal predicament: that so many men still regarded women in general as sexually *inferior*. Others felt resentful and bitter. All of them would have liked to change things. At long last it was no longer my story – it was *our* story.

THE REAL TRUTH ABOUT THE SITUATION

I decided to *act*. At first I had no plan at all. I simply read more sex manuals, ploughed through page after page of women's sexual 'confessions', sought out statistics, and laboured over the po-faced prose of scores of sexologists. I read feminists, sociologists, anthropologists, ethnologists, biologists and plain old doctors. I went to clinics and self-help groups, even if they were only vaguely related to the topic in question, and I steered the conversation round to what interested me.

I was astonished: the women I had talked to in the restaurant were only the tip of the iceberg. The picture that was emerging was more dramatic still. Every time we turn on the television, open a magazine or pass a bookshop sex stares us in the face. Facts about sex, stories, advice and techniques. The overall impression is that every adult – and a good many children, come to that – in the western world is highly educated about sex, and by extension highly expert in the bedroom. But the truth is that there is still an astonishing level of ignorance about sexual matters. And it makes life unhappy for thousands of men and hundreds of thousands of women.

The more I read and the more I talked, the more I appreciated just how vast a body of women needed help, either to climax *whenever* they wanted, or to climax at all. And, I should add, how vast a body of men needed educating.

Then I discovered *The Hite Report*. Hite's statistics reveal that of her volunteer sample only 30 per cent have an orgasm regularly from intercourse. Twenty-nine per cent have never reached orgasm during intercourse. The rest lie somewhere in between. A later survey of 4000 British respondents to *Woman* magazine came up with an even lower figure. I was shocked and (I have to admit) a little pleased – there's nothing like solidarity in adversity to improve your spirits.

Furthermore it's a pretty safe guess that the statistics are worse than that. Because if it's a volunteer sample, the women most likely to come forward and be candid about sex are likely to be those who are also successful with sex. And while many people might be tempted to pretend they *do* orgasm when they *don't*, few are likely to pretend that they *don't* when they *do*. That's about as probable as a woman claiming she weighs ten stone when she actually weighs nine.

These revelations left me feeling dizzy. It was Christmas time, and everyone else seemed very jolly. I remember wandering listlessly about my flat, vaguely trying to pin the fairy on the Christmas tree and thinking that perhaps, after all, women weren't meant to have orgasms. Never mind the Nativity story, all I could think of was the Old Testament: Genesis, Adam and Eve, The

Fall. That's it! I decided. The Bible was right; it's all true really. This is God's punishment for Eve and that beastly apple. I took the fairy off the tree and hung up a snake instead.

Two days later I had a lucky break.

The first stage of my liberation came on the day I met the Mangaians . . .

THOSE MARVELLOUS MANGAIANS

I remember it well. It was 1981, and I was musing over one of my Christmas presents, a bumper illustrated Royal Wedding Album given to me by a well-meaning aunt. Weddings, I thought – honeymoons – sex – orgasms. Do royalty have orgasms? I wondered. Shall I write to the Queen and ask her?

My speculations were interrupted by the sound of my boyfriend wolfing down his beans on toast. He had done himself proud the night before and climaxed twice in under an hour. Now we sat at breakfast the morning after, me picking dejectedly at a croissant, while he congratulated himself.

Before you start thinking that he must have been a monster of conceit, wait a moment: I *don't* mean that he sat there saying, 'My God, I did it well last night. What a stud I am!' Believe me, if this was the case he wouldn't have been sitting there in one piece for long. What he *actually* said was, 'Mmmm, it was good last night' (leaning over to give me a kiss). 'One of the really great fucks. I feel ready for anything this morning' – all uttered with a charming smile and a (slightly absent-minded) ruffle of my hair. A very typical morning-after scenario, in fact.

The trouble was, I hadn't climaxed at all. We'd been together several months and he seemed very happy with the relationship. Either it never occurred to him to wonder how *I* was enjoying the sex, or, more probably, he didn't really want to hear if I had any complaints and thought it best not to ask. After all, if there was something wrong, wasn't it up to me to mention it?

20

This particular boyfriend was an anthropologist, due off on another trip to darkest Africa. I wasn't especially sorry to see him go. He finished his coffee and went off to have a shower. He'd left some of his books lying around and, idly, I picked one up. In it there was an article about the sexual life and education of the Mangaians.

What I read changed my life: because on Mangaia, Polynesia, all the woman have orgasms all the time.

Mangaia is one of the Cook Islands in the Pacific. It may be a long way off, and it may be small, but the fact is that fundamentally the women there are just the same as you and me. They don't have different anatomies; they don't have orgasmic drugs; they don't undergo hypnosis – the only difference is that in their culture women and men are *trained* to get maximum satisfaction from sex.

Their approach is straightforward. In my more frustrated moments I've often wondered what it would take to get it adopted in all its glory over here. Boys begin their sexual education when they're thirteen or fourteen with an older, experienced woman. She teaches them techniques of foreplay and cunnilingus, skills to be practised briefly and with the sole purpose of arousing the woman sufficiently for coitus. Intercourse lasts – Oh, the bliss of it! – from fifteen to thirty minutes, during which the woman, who has also been trained in sexual proficiency from an early age, climaxes two or three times. The man withholds his orgasm until the very end.

If a man is an unsatisfactory lover the woman may leave him and spread news of his inadequacy throughout the island. He quickly gets a 'reputation', and will then find it hard to get another woman to have sex with him.

This remarkable evidence for the importance of *learning* in sexual relations is to be found by studying the few societies in the world where sexual training is an integral part of the culture. Just recently I was reading about a similar community in the Himalayas called the Lachas, and another one in the South Seas – there, too, all the women have orgasms during sex.

I was thrilled to bits. It seemed just the omen I needed to reverse my gloomy thoughts. Of course I was well aware that my lifestyle and upbringing were a world away from that of the Mangaians. But their story convinced me that given the right training, *any* woman can *learn* to have an orgasm. *They gave me the confidence to start training myself*. There and then I began to devise my plan. I have never looked back . . .

CHAPTER THREE

OUR STORY – SUCCESS

So, if you have trouble with orgasm you now know that many of the women you see when you walk down the street are in the same boat, although they'd be loath to admit it.

The mistake that is so often made, however, is to assume that your ability to have an orgasm is simply a personal characteristic which you've got to accept willy-nilly, like having a big nose or short legs. So many women worry that they cannot do it because they weren't born that sort of person, or because there was some quality in their upbringing that upset their chances for ever.

This is rubbish. Not only the Mangaians, but science, theory and practice all show that women can *learn* to have an orgasm.

WOMEN AS THE SUBTLER SEX

It has long been known that whereas a man's orgasm is a simple affair, a woman's orgasm is much more sophisticated. It has nothing to do with failure or inadequacy, it is simply a feature of our existence. In evolutionary terms men *have* to climax quickly. If, several hundred thousand years ago, they weren't able to produce a pretty nippy ejaculation they probably would have been eaten by a sabre-toothed tiger, and the human race would've died out.

Unfortunately for women, the survival of the species never depended on *their* climaxing at all. One of the really fascinating things about female orgasms – or maddening, depending on your point of view – is that nobody really knows *why* they happen at all. And if nobody knows why they happen, it's hardly surprising that we can't agree why they *don't* happen.

In Chapter 16 I discuss the different theories that specialists have devised to account for the existence of female orgasm. Suffice here to say that the great gulf between men's ready ability and women's difficulty has not been helped by the fact that, even in our advanced, sexually 'enlightened' era, ignorance of women's sexual needs still predominates. Researchers are constantly amazed and fascinated by the great sexual potential of women. Too many women – precisely because of the complexity of their sexuality – do not appreciate how to make use of these qualities. And, perhaps more importantly, too many men do not appreciate it either.

Scientists agree that in evolutionary terms a woman's orgasm is much more advanced than a man's. In the females of most lower species, it is absent. But whatever polemical point you want to make about this, no one can deny that it *is* interesting, and it sheds an enormous glare of light on the problem of why women have more difficulty with orgasms than men. The male and female orgasms may be similar sensations, but they represent very different degrees of sophistication.

WHAT'S WRONG WITH ME? NOTHING!

Whatever your reason for wanting an easy orgasm, or just any orgasm during sex – be it personal satisfaction, to prove a point or just out of interest – this book can help you to achieve it. However much we are told not to worry about failure to climax, orgasm-related anxieties will not vanish, any more than dieting-related anxieties vanish because we are told we should 'learn to live with ourselves'.

The terms 'frigid' and 'cold' may have disappeared from the sex books, but unfortunately many women are still tormented with them. I recently read in a popular women's magazine of a sixteen-year-old girl who, after having had sex for the first time with her 'experienced' boyfriend, was taunted about being 'frigid' because she found it painful and distressing. Or, as one married woman commented to me, 'What a crazy, ironic description. Here I am lying in bed, almost *boiling over* with frustration, and he calls me *cold*.'

After the sex researchers finally realized that these labels were not only nasty, but scientifically untenable, they congratulated themselves on the introduction of a new term: 'dysfunctional'. Not a great improvement, but a small step forward. To my mind it still manages to capture most of the unpleasant overtones of the old words, but dilutes them a little with the cold objectivity of science. It's a term divided into two parts: 'primary' or 'secondary'. If you've never had an orgasm then, says the sexologist, you have a 'primary dysfunction'. If you've sometimes had one, but less than 50 per cent of the time, then you've only got 'secondary dysfunction'. In my case when I began my self-help programme I was resoundingly 'primary'.

But things are changing again. Because now, in answer to that nagging question 'What's wrong with me?', scientists are finally beginning to realize that the answer is 'Nothing'. Moreover, since it is the great majority of women – something like 70 per cent – who have trouble achieving orgasm, it is simply inaccurate to consider them abnormal. As the English sexologist Martin Cole recently wrote, 'The terms "frigid" and "dysfunctive" when applied to women who do not achieve orgasm are simply "intellectually unacceptable".' It makes no more sense than to label the minority of people who practise (for example) foot fetishism 'normal' and the rest of us who prefer plain old sexual intercourse 'deviants'. Women who were once called 'frigid' and more recently 'orgasmically dysfunctive' actually have nothing wrong with them at all. All that's the matter is that they have not yet been able to develop fully their orgasmic skills.

So let's get rid of those repressive old terms like 'abnormal', 'failure' and 'inadequacy', and start thinking about our sexual state as being 'pre-orgasmic' – a term that is gradually becoming accepted in the scientific world. It's not only more pleasant, but it's also scientifically more accurate to do so. You are no more an 'abnormal' person because you have not yet learned to make the most of your sexual potential than you were 'abnormal' before you learned the skills of reading and writing, riding a bicycle, playing a musical instrument, painting a picture or speaking a foreign language. Just as you learned these sophisticated skills, so you must *learn*, by means of simple, easy-to-follow exercises, to have an orgasm.

WHY ARE SOME WOMEN PRE-ORGASMIC AND NOT OTHERS?

This question is, of course, the one that everybody would like to be able to answer. As with many sciences, in sexology ignorance is the general rule. I am not being flippant or damning. The average person thinks of science as all-powerful: it takes a physicist to tell you just how *little* is known about the universe, what a small drop of certainty our knowledge really amounts to.

So it is with sexology. The fact remains that for all the shelves full of sexology manuals – and I have ploughed through a good many of these – there are vast areas which nobody adequately understands. And women's sexual response is particularly difficult to monitor – not least because we don't have the erection to give out loud and clear signals of our arousal and climax.

In fact reading about the methods of early researchers and their primitive devices for measuring female response is quite entertaining. Shortly after the First World War, a sexologist, John B. Watson, decided that sex was too important to be left to the medical profession and devised his own set of instruments. Watson connected his own body and that of his female partner to his very primitive equipment while they made love, and produced what were quite likely the very first reliable data on human sexual responses which he catalogued carefully in a set of boxes. But the story ended dramatically when his wife discovered why her husband was spending so much time in his laboratory. She sued for divorce and confiscated all his scientific records. The case made lurid headline news and Watson ended his days in an advertising agency.

Nowadays sexology equipment is sophisticated. But, because there are so many factors influencing our sexual responses, studies tend to concentrate on tiny areas and have small numbers of participants. Almost invariably their conclusions are tentative and likely to be disproved or challenged the following month. Sexologists simply cannot agree.

So it is not surprising to learn that the causes of orgasmic difficulty in women are still not understood. In some cases the partner is not sexually suitable for the woman; in other cases the lover may not know how best to stimulate her clitoral area. But in general difficulty with orgasm is due to a mixture of causes, including psychological ones. What researchers do agree about is that in almost all cases there is no *physical* reason why a woman can't have an orgasm. (Those rare cases when a medical condition is to blame, and what can be done about it, are discussed in Chapter 17.)

In individual cases there can be dominant influences. Fear of inadequacy is a major inhibiting factor that many of us have felt at one time. But surely even women who *do* climax sometimes feel this too? The trouble is, the woman who fails to have an orgasm risks getting into that vicious circle: 'failure', which causes fear of 'failure', which in turn induces anxiety and therefore certain 'failure'.

Some women cannot climax because, deep down, they fear orgasm. They see it as a loss of control, and have even described it as 'having a fit', 'going wild', 'losing hold of myself'. This programme will help to allay such fears, because cultivating a sense of *control* is fundamental to it. Control over your own body,

27

control over your own sexual responses at all stages, even when you are being penetrated by a man. Far from being out of control during orgasm, you will learn to be *in control* as never before.

Perhaps the most overriding belief is that women's lack of orgasm is a legacy of our cultural past, the result of our society's attitudes to women, built up over the centuries. Broadly speaking, our society says that whereas men have powerful 'sex drives' that need satisfying, women do not. More than that, women *should* not. For centuries women have been told that to be anything but passive is dirty, unladylike, altogether undesirable. Because women's orgasms are much more dependent on psychological factors than men's, these causes can have profoundly inhibiting effects which we must learn to overcome.

Even though this repressive attitude is slowly disappearing, its influence is still strong and should not be underrated. It colours women's childhoods in numerous small ways, both at home and at school; it is reflected in the media, in endless social conventions – each of which appears insignificant when considered on its own, but which in total has a devastating effect – and it colours men's attitude to women in the bedroom. If women's orgasms were as straightforward as men's, these influences would be annoying but not dramatic; but because women's orgasms are complicated and subtle, the influence can be a significant obstacle to the natural learning process.

WHAT TYPE OF WOMAN HAS TROUBLE WITH ORGASM?

Now that we know that the majority of women are to some degree pre-orgasmic, the question of what *type* of woman has trouble becomes increasingly meaningless. Princess to pauper, it affects us all.

Even if we try to narrow the field and ask what type of woman has *great* difficulty with orgasm – the woman, for example, who has never climaxed – it's very hard to pinpoint the answer.

Needless to say hundreds of studies have tried to do just that.

One researcher, for example, concluded that the only consistent factor among women who had trouble with orgasm was the quality of their early relationship with their father: those who perceived him not to have invested a serious or dependable interest in them were more likely to report orgasmic difficulties. There was no such correlation with relationships with mothers. But is this universally the case, or simply the oddity of that particular study? There has been some – undramatic – support for this idea, but as always the conclusions are cautious. Having thought about it in relation to myself, it seems to me credible that the woman who is accustomed to a relaxed, stable relationship with a man might well do better in bed.

I'd always believed that women with repressively religious upbringings had difficulty with orgasm, because of inherent guilt, and also that women who've undergone trauma, such as rape or incest, would have trouble climaxing. But, according to a number of detailed studies, there is no evidence for either association. In 1966, in an unpublished doctoral dissertation mentioned in Fisher, D. F. Shope even discovered that, in the sample investigated, unmarried orgasmic women had *more* traumatic sexual encounters before the age of sixteen than their non-orgasmic counterparts. The sexologist Seymour Fisher also claims that education has some influence – better educated women have a little less trouble than their uneducated sisters, although this may be because educated women demand more from their lovers and are less content to settle for second best. My favourite result is that of a group of researchers who discovered that church-going English women tended to have less trouble with orgasm than the impious ladies who went elsewhere on Sunday – sure suggestion that hell's delights might not be so great after all.

Among all the many women I've spoken to I've never come across a 'type' of woman who has difficulty with orgasm. It is a problem which affects rich women and poor, successful and unsuccessful, thin and fat, glamorous and homely, healthy and unhealthy, old and young.

All in all, the only really predictable factor is the diversity!

DOES THERAPY HELP?

Some women may find therapists, psychologists and counsellors helpful regarding sexual difficulties. They didn't work for me at all. And, looking at the results of many women I've known, I tend to be sceptical. Whereas I've heard success stories when it comes to family problems, self-confidence, anxiety and phobias, sex problems can be maddeningly elusive and difficult for the professional to treat. (Besides, whenever I see the word 'therapist' my eye changes it to 'the rapist'.)

My first therapist was nicely mannered, with limp advice and endless euphemisms. 'How can I be sure of faking my orgasm successfully so that my boyfriend won't start calling me "frigid"?' I asked her innocently one day. Ms Therapist almost fell backwards off her chair. She spluttered a bit and then began burbling on about love, honesty and understanding.

'Look' – I *had* to interrupt her – 'I *have* tried that actually. Oddly enough I too like love and understanding in a partnership. But it doesn't always make you come.' I crawled home feeling more than usually guilty about faking, and scared that I was about to be found out.

After her I moved to a stern young man who sat up stiffly as if glued to his seat in the wrong position. Each week I steeled myself to face his grim expression. It didn't encourage me to open up. I soon formed the impression that he was feeling his way in his profession, yet tried to cover this up by being assertive. It did not inspire confidence when I came in one day to find him quickly shuffling a 'How To'-type textbook into his drawer behind a half-eaten Mars Bar. Another of his tricks was to make an elaborate pretence that he wasn't looking at his watch, but was pulling up his shirtsleeves and scratching his wrist. I watched this performance for several weeks before I interrupted him:

'Why don't you just look at the clock on the wall if you want to know the time? Have you any idea how hurtful all that subterfuge is?' After all, it's not easy to talk freely on delicate topics when you are worrying that he is longing for the session to end. When he didn't like what I'd said he simply fell silent, with a Buddha-like smile on his face.

My respect for him really plummeted when I went away on holiday. He knew my hobby was natural history, so I selected a dramatic postcard of a spider to send to him.

When it came to our next session he lay in wait, fingering the postcard.

'I think you want to eat me,' he blurted out.

'*What?*' I replied incredulously.

Immediately his face fell. 'Isn't that what female spiders do? Eat their mates?'

For Christ's sake, I thought, he doesn't even know. Very helpful for my problems.

The worst of all came two weeks before I was due to be 'terminated' (nice expression, that). I'd missed a session because of a crisis at home, but forgotten to telephone him to say so. He jumped to the conclusion that I was 'running away'. The following day a letter arrived in the post, informing me that I had some 'very serious problems' to sort out, and warning me against missing the last two sessions. It seemed astonishing to me that, in my apparently 'fragile' state of mind, he could think fit to taunt me with it.

'What panacea do you think you can offer in two hours that you've failed to do in two years?' I demanded. He, of course, chose to remain silent, nodding his head like one of those plastic Alsatians people used to have in the back of their cars. It was an unnecessary and upsetting end to the therapy, made worse when he informed me that I was 'unable to open up and confront my problems'.

'Yes,' I agreed. 'Unable with you.' I knew this was true because, on several occasions when he'd been ill, I'd felt quite relaxed with his replacement. But he wouldn't admit that. I left with my confidence lower than when I'd started. I see now, with hindsight, just how irresponsible his attitude was. We were mismatched; he preferred to blame me. At the time I was particularly vulnerable and I trusted him. I did not have the self-confidence to get angry, so I grew depressed.

I mention this episode because so often therapy is regarded as a universal cure for all problems. And not enough is said about the frightening way in which an incompetent or even mismatched therapist can do harm.

Of course, this is not to say that psychotherapy cannot be helpful. Although sex researchers have found little evidence to show that it is effective in treating sexual difficulties, some people find the involvement of a third, objective, professional person in their sex life comforting and encouraging. In individual cases, if not in general, psychotherapy can then be useful. If you're lucky enough to be able to get a good therapist, then by all means take advantage of the opportunity.

Behavioural sex therapy, such as that developed by Masters and Johnson, is far more successful. Instead of trying to approach the problem negatively by concentrating on resolving 'inner conflicts' (just what these are depends on the school to which your psychotherapist adheres), the behaviourist takes a positive approach. By informing the woman about the true nature of her sexuality, and by training her physically to make full use of her sexual potential and overcome her inhibitions, these therapists have reported remarkable results. But it is important that you be the right sort of participant in such a programme: if you can afford the fees, and the time it takes, and if you have the peculiar sort of nerve required to go through with such a programme wholeheartedly, *and* if your partner is equally willing (most behaviourists will only treat the couple together), then you might consider it.

There's one other thing, too. Although these therapists have very good results, you've got to keep going. Often after a participant has left the programme, her earlier difficulties slowly return. This is, in my opinion, because the programmes frequently don't concentrate enough on developing the individual woman's capacity to learn. They place too much emphasis on the importance of both partners – an admirable approach, but not always a practical one. Relationships change and outside of the constructive atmosphere of the sex clinic the gains may soon be whittled away.

Personally, I knew I had to do it alone.

CHAPTER FOUR

WOMEN TAKE CONTROL

Women's ability to have an orgasm is a skill which – like all the skills of civilization – we need to develop. All that is required is a willingness to learn. Both women and men will benefit.

I have already stated that there are various possible reasons why women find themselves unable to have an orgasm: our cultural heritage, personal upbringing, lack of adequate stimulation from our partners, and so forth.

To all these I have something important to add – something to which the sex therapists give scant attention: control. I believe that a sense of control is the most important feature in achieving orgasm. By control I do not mean domination: I mean a sense of taking charge of your own life, your own body, and your own orgasm. And control is something that women still do not have enough of – especially in the bedroom.

THE PROBLEM OF THE INVISIBLE BARRIER

Sounds like a Sherlock Holmes story, doesn't it? Let me explain what I mean.

All the while I was agonizing over why I didn't have an orgasm, and trying to develop my training programme, it struck me as particularly significant that almost without exception women can easily achieve orgasm by masturbation. Indeed, the majority of women in sexologist Alfred Kinsey's study masturbated to orgasm within four minutes. Yet most of these same women have difficulty achieving orgasm during intercourse; many of them have great difficulty; and some, like myself before I began training, don't have them at all.

To some extent this vast discrepancy is explained by the fact that the men do their part inadequately. They don't provide their partner with enough stimulation, they ejaculate too quickly, they are too rough, their position is wrong, etc. These are what I call the 'technicalities' of sex and they *are*, of course, very important.

However, this is not a sufficient explanation for women's lack of orgasm. There are many times when the partner is all attention and understanding, but still no go. Susannah's problem is typical:

> This bloke was a god as far as I was concerned. Nice chunky legs and a gorgeous behind that came in at the sides. Strong arms, and a face that made me want to come just to look at it. He was also an excellent lover – gentle, patient and inventive. Did my pussy pay any attention? No it didn't. But the most annoying thing was that as soon as he'd finished (we'd do it for an hour and a half, probably more) leaving me still desperate, all I had to do was pop into the loo and do it to myself in a couple of minutes. Now what foul trick of nature is that?

And quite apart from this, women *should* be able to achieve orgasm even when conditions are not 100 per cent ideal. They can quickly learn to have an orgasm through masturbation even in the most adverse circumstances, as Deborah's story shows:

> My masturbation techniques are quite crude and unimaginative really – I realize that since reading *Hite*. Just a short rub *anywhere* around there, it doesn't even have to be on target, and I come. Yet Vince, who really has a lot more patience and skill, has to work for a *long long* time before

I can even think of coming. Even then it's only about 50
per cent success.

What happened between Deborah's own sexual attentions to
herself, and the attentions of her boyfriend? *What happened* between
Susannah's own sexual attentions to herself, and the attentions of
her boyfriend? The story is the same for thousands of women. A
barrier appeared; an *invisible* but powerful one. This invisible barrier
is a maddening phenomenon. Perfectly ordinary women with no
physical or psychological handicaps are simply not able to have an
orgasm during sex, for no apparent reason.

How do we explain it? I believe the answer is that this invisible barrier represents a *loss of control*. In both Susannah's and
Deborah's cases it was not simply a technical difference between
masturbation and sex with their partner – it was the difference
between having total control over the situation and having only
partial control. For many women, the sense of 'another' is deeply,
perhaps unconsciously, disturbing. We do not readily allow
another person to 'control' us. Especially when that 'other' is
engaged in something as intimate as sexual stimulation.

When I began devising this plan I realized an important truth
about myself: I had only really begun to enjoy sex when I'd
realized that the man did not have to be sexually dominant. In
other words, the more control I gained in the bedroom, the closer
it brought me to satisfying sex, to overcoming this pernicious
invisible barrier.

In my case this came to me as part of my growing confidence as
I got older. Before then I had had good times and bad times in
bed. I had certainly got sexually aroused. But I had rarely felt
totally *at ease*. There was always the feeling that the man led and I
followed. I didn't want to follow and I didn't particularly want to
lead. *I wanted to be equal*.

I began to analyse why my early sexual encounters were so
unsatisfying. With experience I had achieved a greater degree of
co-ordination of the situation. I was less a 'subject' of my partner,
more psychologically comfortable with him, less self-consciously
aware that he was a 'separate', potentially critical, individual.

And, of course, I was more confident of making sure that he pleased me as much as I pleased him.

I discovered that among my friends it was often the older women who had more success with sex. Several had had a bad time of it when young, but later had managed to find satisfaction, or at least to get a good bit closer to achieving orgasm. And the reason? Because these older women had learned to get over their youthful worries and insecurities. They were more at ease with their sexuality and more confident of themselves.

This feeling of lack of control during sex is difficult to pin down in words. Think hard about your own situation and you will begin to understand what I am driving at. In fact, I use the word 'driving' advisedly, because the most helpful analogy I can make is that of learning familiarity with a motor car. When you begin to learn how to drive, you feel like you are holding the steering wheel of a malicious-minded metal dinosaur. It seems as if at any moment the car might simply decide to stop paying attention to you, and do something silly of its own accord. Getting from A to B seems rather a matter of luck. Gradually you become more and more familiar with the beast, until that marvellous moment, usually long after you have passed your driving test, when you realize that *you* have complete control of the car, not the other way around. Gone is that element of chance in how the car moves: you have really mastered it.

This applies to anything else you have learned to do successfully – ride a bicycle, operate a word processor, bake a cake, even look after a baby. That feeling of *total* control, total *ease*, a professional sense of what you are doing, is what you are aiming for sexually. Not in regard to your partner, but in regard to yourself and your partner*ship*.

A sense of control is a vital factor in women's sexual fulfilment. Yet so many women lose control in the bedroom – often without realizing it. In fact, the idea of control is so important that, although the distinctions are not watertight and sometimes overlap, I have divided it into two types: Visible Control and Invisible Control.

Visible Control

The first kind of control you will learn in the programme is 'Visible Control'. I call it that because it is control over the visible, tangible parts of yourself: your own body and its responses. You will train your body, step-by-step, to respond sexually. At the end you will know precisely *what you like* and what you don't – regardless of what sex books tell you is enjoyable. Barbara gives a good example of this:

> How many times have I read in books that earlobes are erogenous zones! So I thought, OK. I let men keep on at them, hating every minute but thinking I must be odd. I thought if I kept on maybe I'll start to like it. It made me wince.
>
> At long last I realized: that's not me. I had the confidence to say no, I hate it and I'll always hate it and it doesn't matter in the least. Because what I do like is having the back of my neck nibbled. If that's odd – I don't give a damn.

Sex will no longer be a 'lie back and hope for the best' affair as it was for Rosalind, who

> just used to think that if I could only really relax, let the guy take over, it'd all be OK. Relax, relax, relax – my counsellor used to use that word ad nauseum. She said I was 'fighting' sex and must learn to relax. I used to twist myself in knots trying to relax. I relaxed so much I went to sleep. I felt it was a mistake for me to try and guide him, and that I should gracefully accept what he did and not change it. Well, I kept this up for two years and it got me just *nowhere*. 'Lie back and relax' is *the* biggest sex myth.

Nor will it be a 'try everything and hope for the best' business as it was for Phillipa:

> **After I realized I had problems with orgasm I thought it
> was because I was too dull. Every book I picked up showed
> couples doing outrageous things to each other and having
> wild orgasms. I really did believe that if I could be more
> adventurous I would succeed. I was completely wrong; in
> fact I hated it most of the time. I can tell you, categorically
> now, the *only* way to enjoy fancy sex is after you've really
> mastered the basics. I just wish someone had told me that
> years ago.**

Rosalind and Phillipa are right. In learning to have an orgasm
every time you want one it is *not* enough to lie back, relax and let
the man take over. Nor is it a wise move to be shamed by advanced
sex manuals into exotic options. The way to permanent, constant
success with orgasm is gradually and carefully – with you taking a
major role.

Invisible Control

Invisible Control is something more subtle and elusive – a state of
mind, which means it's harder to pin down.

I think we are all getting familiar with the ways in which, in
ordinary life, so-called equality for men and women can mask a
range of inequalities. For example, women have won the right to
enter previously male professions such as medicine and the law;
they have won the right to equal pay and, theoretically, to equal
prospects. Where they exist, these are clearly defined 'equalities'.
Now we have to tackle all the subtleties of inequality that legisla-
tion cannot handle: the fact that in many of these jobs women
must be twice as good to be accepted, that again and again they
get passed over for promotion; that undermining sexual harass-
ment still goes unchecked. Angelica Huston put it well when,
shortly after the release of *The Addams Family*, she was interviewed
by *Hello!* magazine:

'You have said before that women are trained to yield to men, to defer to them, so to speak. Is this true in your case?' they asked.

'Well,' she replied, 'it's not so much about yielding, it's more a sort of acquiescence, like this is more important for him than it is for me. I just won't do that, but women feel that in order to be feminine they can't be aggressive, and it's a fine line.'

Now translate these kinds of attitudes to the bedroom. Again and again in sexual situations female equality is seen as female stridency – by the women themselves, often as not.

To begin with, what I have described as Invisible Control is not feeling yourself duty bound to place his needs before yours.

'Well, that's obvious,' the more enlightened readers might protest. I thought it was obvious too – but all the time I am realizing just how difficult that is to put into practice. In fact my own views were very similar to those of Veronica:

> I think of myself as utterly liberated – in *everything*. And yet so often I catch myself making little concessions to his pleasure in bed. I feel I have to give his genitals more attention than he gives mine. If he's getting really excited and close to orgasm I feel I oughtn't to stop him so that I can catch up – I let him go right ahead and enjoy himself – and so I'm left frustrated. And, even when he *does* give me lots of attention, I often feel slightly guilty, as if I'm having a treat, not something that's due to me. It's almost as if these responses are programmed into me. When I notice them, I get very angry with myself – yet I find it hard to stop and really enforce my equality.

Again and again I have listened to this response from women – I quote only Veronica precisely because the others are so similar. I too believe passionately in women's rights – but it is not a feminist obsession to recognize that women are encouraged from birth to be second to men *sexually*. This is an impression I have built up over years of speaking to both men and women. To make the point I quote here a selection of men I have recently interviewed.

> I have to admit that however forceful a woman is outside the bedroom, they're usually pretty accommodating in. All the women I've been to bed with just lie there and wait for me to get on with it. I wish they wouldn't. The only exception that I can recall is a French girl I met in Paris.

> Goodness, I wish women *would* be more assertive. It's sexy. [This man was laconic – he blushed and wouldn't say any more.]

And the only one out of twenty who showed a definite preference for 'passive' women:

> Thank God, yes, women seem to have an inbuilt sense that men come first in the bedroom. Even aggressive ones? Yeee-ees . . . yes, definitely. In fact the only woman I've ever bedded who was bossy in bed was pretty low-key outside. Must have been. If I'd guessed I wouldn't have seduced her!

However, the real difficulty of sexual equality in the bedroom is that of *identifying* it in the first place. This vague but undermining feeling of sexual submissiveness – of not feeling fully in control in a relationship – creeps in in all sorts of insidious ways, however 'liberated' we feel. As Veronica (above) has made clear, it takes sensitivity and vigilance to spot our inequalities and a great deal of self-confidence to eradicate them.

A lot of different factors combine to give women a bad start in sexual equality. Firstly, the ease with which men can have an orgasm means that many women feel themselves less sexually capable, and therefore something of a sexual underling by comparison. (It is precisely this feeling that this book seeks to redress.) It is for the woman that the man waits; it is for the woman that he extends his foreplay, etc. *He* doesn't need these things for himself. Because women are sexually more sophisticated they take longer to warm up and they require more skilled lovemaking than men. In fact, many sexologists believe that a woman's lack of orgasm simply reflects the man's incapacity to retain his semen.

Secondly, men often *are* more sexually experienced. This doesn't mean simply that they've had more partners, but that they, finding sex so much more readily gratifying, have quickly learned how to make the most of it. A recent article in *Woman's Own* revealed that 48 per cent of girls have had sexual intercourse before the age of sixteen. Almost invariably these early sexual encounters are more pleasurable for the male than for the female. The race for sexual satisfaction has begun and already men have a head-start. It can take years for a woman to catch up.

Sex manuals don't help much either. Many women have pointed out to me that the one picture they could remember from sex guides was how to rub a man's penis, or how to suck him off. This is partly because women's genitals are smaller, more discreet than men's (or, like the clitoris, hardly visible at all). Cunnilingus is usually a picture of a man's head with a little twizzle of pubic hair poking out around his mouth. But fellatio is a huge phallus, 'rubbing his penis' is a huge phallus, and 'delaying ejaculation with your finger and thumb' ditto. Small things on their own, but they add to the general feeling that the man is the more important partner. The very size and visibility of a man's sexual parts compared to the discreet female genitalia has an effect. When we look at old Greek vase paintings of erotic scenes, the men have huge erections and give the obvious impression of 'feeling horny'. As for the women, whatever position they are in, how can we tell if they are highly aroused?

Economic factors also play a part in limiting women's sense of control in the bedroom. Many women feel that they must put their partner's sexual needs before their own or they will lose him. As long as women are economically dependent upon men – which with children they often cannot help but be – this situation will continue. As one mother of four told me, 'I don't enjoy my husband's lovemaking. But what can I do? If he goes off I'm left with four kids, no money and little prospect of attracting another partner. Looked at like that bad sex is a small price to pay.'

Another reason for loss of control in the bedroom is that during sex we are always keeping half a mind on how we look, constantly asking, 'Am I alluring enough between the sheets? Slim enough? Pretty enough?' And, of course, 'Am I a good lover?' But most of the men, when I asked them, said they only worried about such things at the very beginning of a relationship. Just the simple fact of being able to walk around the bedroom naked and unembarrassed, as men always seem able to do, gives them an advantage. So many women, anxious to look 'perfect' for their lover, feel they must grab a dressing gown to hide their 'defects'. The fact that the man may not mind these 'defects' doesn't make much difference. A recent survey in *Woman* magazine revealed that a massive 84 per cent of women believe they are too fat. Translate that to the bedroom, where we cannot hide behind a well-tailored jacket or a loose skirt, and you can begin to calculate the damage to women's self-esteem.

Countless studies have shown that men have a far more positive self-image than women. For example, when a group of people were asked to comment on their physical attractiveness, almost unanimously the women tended to describe themselves in terms of their defects – 'My bottom's too large', 'I'd like to change my mouth' and so forth – while the men described themselves in relation to their positive points – 'I have good legs, nice hair' etc. The *Woman* survey also revealed the astonishing and somewhat tragic fact that only 7 per cent of women are confident enough to want to look like no one but themselves – Princess Diana, Victoria Principal and Yasmin Le Bon being the top three preferred ideals. Of course this kind of self-doubt takes its toll in the bedroom.

There is also the much-held popular view that whereas a woman is content with one partner for many years, men need a variety of lovers to keep their interest. This 'seven-year itch' has been the subject of numerous films – most famously that of the same name in which Marilyn Monroe plays a (guess what?) curvaceous blonde tempting a man away from his staid wife. So that for many women the very time when after several years with their partner they should be feeling most at ease physically and emotionally, they are also beginning to worry that their partner will tire of them.

Before you begin to wonder whether you wouldn't rather go and take the dog for a walk than read all this gloom and doom, let me stress that I am not necessarily talking about what *is* – but about the kind of things women *fear*. The very fact of recognizing such things is the first step to eradicating them.

Outside the bedroom there is another undermining factor which can cause you to feel loss of control in a sexual sense. This is the feeling of being the 'prey' of a man, under his scrutiny. Still it is men who are usually the ones to seek out, size up and make proposals to women. However high our self-confidence, an aggressive pick-up approach can make us feel less of an individual, more of an anonymous female.

My friend Letitia had had a bad experience with a sexually domineering partner. Fortunately she found an excellent – and unexpected – way of getting round her feelings of loss of control. She was invited to Epsom to watch the Derby, but became separated from her party. Longing for some refreshment, and finding all the tables occupied, she sat down next to a single young man. He, some years younger than she, looked quiet and nervous; after a while they began talking. He invited her for a drink, and then – somewhat abashed at his own boldness – to supper, which he didn't have enough money to pay for, so they split the bill. With most men she would have been on guard right from the start, but this one seemed to have to muster up so much courage for each stage of his courtship that she felt not in the least bit threatened by it. As she said, 'He was not one to start lungeing, and even if he had it wouldn't have taken much to push him off.' Back at her flat he lost his nerve. He was charming, intelligent, nice looking, and Letitia really began to fancy him, but he was rooted to the spot for fear of affronting her with any bold advances. So in the end she leaned over and kissed him . . .

I can still remember the surprise I felt and the liberation. Even when we were lying together making love in the most ordinary manner possible I felt that the whole scene was containable. He was the one doing the worrying; if I was not satisfied he would feel it must be his fault, not mine. And because he was so obviously young, nervous and inexperienced I didn't have the feeling that I was under scrutiny. I had no intention of making him feel submissive, but I relished his complete inability to behave dominantly. Clearly he had no inherent assumption of his superiority. I knew I could encourage him to satisfy me; my pleasure was no longer accidental.

Letitia's story describes well the importance of sex in which the woman feels relaxed and not under scrutiny. Of course this does not have to be a situation in which she is dominant:

The trouble for me was that I wanted more than anything for Mark to fling me down on the bed and force me to have sex with him while he held my arms back. I loved the feeling of being pushed around during sex. But I didn't want to also submit my enjoyment to his. If he came, then I wanted to come too. As far as having an orgasm was concerned I wanted to be an equal – in that sense, yes, I wanted control. I didn't want to feel that my pleasure was inferior to his, just the sex-role that I played. After I'd got Mark to understand that, everything was dandy. We have plenty of 'male dominance' scenarios together. But I never feel subordinated in my mind. It may be a subtle difference, but it's very important.

In a recent study (Garcia) carried out amongst American college students, an erotic story describing a male and a female engaging in sexual activity was presented to them. The female subjects 'reported more sexual arousal and less negative effect when the female character was described as dominant'. Another researcher, with the charmingly appropriate name of Heiman (sexologists these days have *delightful* names – Seamen, Horney and Hyman Rodman to name just three) found that 'a female-initiated, female-centred narrative was significantly more arousing for female subjects than any of the other variations'.

The sense of being 'prey' to a man is something that many women live with day after day. Let me give you a different example. For years I was hugely flattered whenever a workman wolf-whistled at me, yet I also felt an uncomfortable sense of threat. Then, in my thirties, I grew less obsessed with my appearance and began going out deliberately unmade-up, wearing comfortable (some would say frumpy) clothes. After the initial disappointment of passing a building site in silence and not drawing the occasional admiring glance down the street, I began to see the power of it. For the first time I felt like a real person, not simply a being who existed only in relation to other people's views of me. Sheila Kitzinger quotes a woman who, because of being pregnant, was no longer regarded as a viable sex object:

> **Strangely, once I was no longer bombarded with sexual advances, it struck me how in one way it gave me a sense of power, of attractiveness, and, more importantly, a sense that I existed.**

Germaine Greer's sharp and inspirational *The Change* tells how on a trip to Sicily she decided, as an expression of mourning for her father, to dress in black with her hair covered.

> **I found the new freedom from men's attentions exhilarating rather than depressing. There was also tremendous liberation in not having to think what to wear. Black goes with black. One has only to think of textures, of the part of one's clothing that matters to oneself.**

Of course we all like to feel we *can* look attractive for the right person, or when we *want* to draw admiring glances. But this 'invisible' independence can be, I now realize, a far more powerful feeling than the 'power' of sexual attractiveness. Try it some time

– I'm sure you'll appreciate my point. Most importantly, it helps build up that all-important sense of *control*.

Try to familiarize yourself with Visible Control and Invisible Control – each will have some special meaning to you and your relationship. Once you are conscious of the little ways in which we lose control in sexual relationships, you'll be on the way to helping yourself. The plan has been specially formulated to take them both into account. It works by making use of all the best of the 'technicalities' of sex, while at the same time breaking down the invisible barrier step by step. Taking more control is, therefore, *prescribed*.

THE MYTH OF THE PASSIVE WOMAN

I want to end this chapter on what I think is a particularly cheerful note.

I have talked about our cultural heritage, which has for so long seen women as sexually passive, and how for all the sexual liberation of the 1990s, the myth that women are – or should be – essentially passive still exists. Indeed, I'm a good example of it myself. In my family a woman could be all sorts of things – confident, pushy, career-minded, she could yell at a man in an argument, refuse to do the cooking, slam the door in his face. What she could never do was be sexually forward. If a woman asked a man out, or made the first move, she was considered 'cheap'. I'm in my thirties, but the old Victorianism lingers on. In a sense it's hardly surprising. I've got a copy of the celebrated sex researcher Krafft-Ebing's *Psychopathia Sexualis*, dated 1931 and recommended as a textbook for the medical and legal professions. It states:

> Woman, however, if physically and mentally normal and properly educated, has but little sexual desire.

'Oh,' you may protest, 'that's sixty-three years ago. No wonder it sounds old-fashioned.' Not at all. Both my parents were growing up at that time. 'Old-fashioned' ideas pass easily down the generations and die slowly, very slowly. The new ones hit the headlines and the more outré cinema screens, but the old ones live on for a long time after.

Take a look at so many books and films and you'll see that true romance and love still belongs to the woman who is – in the last analysis – submissive to the man. She may have had oh-so-many adventures/tantrums/escapades/revolts – but when she settles down with the man it's well understood who's actually boss. To take a recent example, the film *Working Girl* purports to portray the modern American woman's rise to power. What happens? Lo and behold, it ends with two women fighting over a man. Mills and Boon sell millions of books worldwide. In every one – at least of the many I've read – the woman, after a period of revolt or individuality, ends up more or less subservient to a dominant man. In many cases he's offensively dominant, almost to the point of rape (only avoided because she 'enjoys it really').

The trouble is, outside of the celluloid, fictional world the passive woman is usually not so lucky. For one thing, it's a serious impediment to achieving orgasm. Lack of control over one's lovemaking leaves you no time to be free to relax, enjoy sex and make sure it satisfies *you*.

And never confuse refusal to be 'passive' with being loud, aggressive and 'unfeminine'. I personally think the limited notions of what is acceptable 'feminine' behaviour are laughable. After all, strong dominant women can be as hugely attractive as frail feminine men. But that is not my point. You can be as firm and insistent as you like, as quietly as you like. In fact quiet insistence, or refusal to give in or compromise, is often the most effective.

Now that I've made my point about refusing to be sexually *passive* – what will your partner think?

'I couldn't possibly be more assertive sexually,' said several women I've spoken to. 'Men hate women like that.'

I used to think so too. In fact, as I've said, it was the mainstay of my upbringing.

Now listen to this.

I *hate* making sexual advances. It makes me feel vulgar and crude.

I usually make the initial sexual advance. How do I feel about it? *I feel precisely that I am less desirable to the woman than she is to me*; and fairly often I feel I'm frightening her. That is one hell of a way to begin. When the woman does make the sexual advance, that alone gives me very positive feelings.

I almost always make the initial sexual advance in all my relationships and I hate it! I feel like I am stealing something or forcing her to do something she may in fact not want to do.

I have a lot of trouble making the initial sexual advance. If I think about it long enough I always come up with enough doubt to keep me from doing anything.

As you've probably gathered by now, these are all men speaking. They come from *The Hite Report on Male Sexuality* and there are scores more. I begin by quoting Hite precisely so that you will *know* I am not making this point to suit my own purposes. In fact Hite identifies the main male complaints about sex as first that women don't want sex often enough, and secondly that *women are too passive*. She shows that, while there are always exceptions, a major sexual dissatisfaction among men is that women do not take the initiative, or participate eagerly: in short, show a degree of control.

After Hite had ascertained men's objections, she asked outright: 'Do men want women to make the first advance?' Here are just three of the responses:

A very aggressive approach by my wife would really be great. For example, if she were to unzip me and pull out my genitals and start to play with them or if she would start undressing me, I would love it.

I'd love to be a sex object at least for a while. I think I'd probably have a heart attack if some woman said to me, 'You turn me on and I'd like to make love with you.'

I often wish they'd be more up-front and tell me what they have in mind. I wonder if they tell Redford in advance.

Hite concludes that while 'only a handful of men said they always preferred to be the aggressors . . . *Over and over again . . . men said they wished the woman would make the first advance.*'

Have *you* ever seduced a man? By which I *don't* mean have you led him on to seducing you – 'I chased her till she caught me,' as some wit once remarked. I mean have you ever been in a situation with a man where you had the upper hand? Have you ever felt *really* in control of the evening, from the moment you stepped out of the front door to the moment you fell asleep beside him? It's a wonderful, heady feeling. And believe me, it works wonders for your sexual ability.

PART TWO

CHAPTER FIVE

PREPARING FOR ORGASM

The only thing you really need to prepare for my programme is one vital ingredient: *yourself*.

This chapter outlines a few considerations that will complement your training programme. It is a long chapter not because there is a lot to do, but because every woman's requirements will be different.

HOW DOES THE PLAN FIT INTO MY LIFE?

The first thing to decide is exactly how you will relate the plan to your normal sex life.

You can, if you like, take a drastic approach and call a halt to your normal mode of operations while you follow the plan through step by step without interruption. This is the approach that most sex clinics would require if you chose to join a professional programme. It is also, to my mind, the least productive and most awkward.

One of the great virtues of this plan is that it does not have a rigid structure, and you should make absolutely sure that you do not feel under pressure from yourself or your partner to get it over and done with as quickly as possible.

A much more profound approach is *gradually* to *replace* your ordinary sex life with stages from the plan. To put it another way, by the end of the plan your new sex life will have replaced the old, but in the meantime you must concentrate on bringing them closer together.

I have said that this plan is suitable for every type of woman – those who have been in long-term relationships as much as those who change their partner regularly. The long-term partnership will probably have the advantage of a greater sense of ease between you and less impatience to 'get on with it'. On the other hand, if you are in a sexual rut (excuse the pun) you may find it difficult to initiate such a programme. The method that the more routine-bound women who tested this plan found worked best was to make a number of different changes. If all kinds of new beginnings gradually start taking place in your life, then sexual change will not stand out so glaringly to your partner. Just about anything at all can fit into this category, depending on your circumstances: a new job, beginning voluntary work, a refreshing holiday, enrolling in evening classes, a new style of dressing, redecorating the house. Then, into the whirlpool of small changes you can introduce sexual change.

HOW LONG WILL THE PLAN TAKE?

If this were a magazine I'd tick you off for being impatient. But how well I understand the desire to see quick results. The best answer I can give you is: it depends. On your partner, on the circumstances, on the point you have reached before you begin the programme, etc. But principally it depends on you. As with dieting, every woman is different and it would be dishonest to try and put a time on any part of this programme. Sooner or later, if you work consistently, you can make the break. One woman I know went from never having had an orgasm to a state where she could succeed 60 per cent of the time in just four weeks. Others have taken the same time just to complete step 3.

But there is one thing I can guarantee: every small success will feel like an enormous breakthrough and will increase your confidence tenfold. To talk of the pleasure of learning may sound corny but in this case it's also true. In the context of a good relationship, each small success is infinitely more intimate than if you'd both been able to do it perfectly from the start. And if you change your partners regularly, these pleasures will be all yours. *That I promise*.

YOUR WORRIES AND GRIEVANCES: ACKNOWLEDGE THEM

Because your sexual success is dependent to a large degree on your mental state, it is important to do whatever you can to build up your self-esteem and rid yourself of anxieties. Of course, what you find most suitable will depend on your own personality and state of confidence. But there are a number of possibilities and factors which you should bear in mind.

When you begin this programme it is a good idea to draw up a list of your worries and grievances about sex. If you are really honest you may find the list gets very long indeed. I know mine was. Don't be disheartened, because by the simple fact of acknowledging that anxieties exist you have taken the first step to curing them. In fact you may find it helpful also to make a list of the things that you particularly enjoy about sex. You can then learn to maximize these.

Pay particular attention to what you feel might be inequalities in your sex life. Perhaps your partner frequently demands a blow job, but is unwilling to give you oral sex in return. Maybe he likes to come quickly, but doesn't put enough effort into your own satisfaction.

The following are just a few examples of what might appear on your list:

I feel uncomfortable making love with the light on
I dislike the look of my partner's penis
My partner always hurries through sex
I worry that he wants to get it over with

I worry that I'm not thin enough
I worry about not having enough lubrication
I always feel very slightly manipulated by him
I can never fully relax during sex, unless I am tipsy

Once you've made the list, start to describe each of the entries in more detail. For example, if you have written 'I dislike the look of my partner's penis', try to pin-point what it is that displeases you. Is it really the penis itself, or is it perhaps the way your partner uses it? If he is pushy and aggressive about his lovemaking, a penis can seem a very threatening object indeed. Or is it that you don't like the feel or taste of it in your mouth?

Try and figure out the strengths and emphases of your worries and think how they might have originated. Give them an order of importance, and consider how to minimize their influence. If there are things that your partner insists upon but that you don't like, decide that at least for the duration of this plan *you will not do them*.

This may not be easy. But now is the time to make a stand. Be *strong* in telling your partner that you don't want to do sex in such and such a way: don't apologize, and don't be surly about it. Just be firm. Haughty, if you like. As one male friend of mine remarked:

> **There is actually something terribly sexy about a woman making it quite clear she knows what she wants and what she doesn't want. It makes her seem unattainable, not to be taken for granted, and therefore doubly desirable. I'd far rather have a woman who pleasantly told me in no uncertain terms that she *hated* performing oral sex, than one who submitted grudgingly.**

It's amazing how your own enjoyment of sex can increase simply by eliminating the pressure to do something you don't particularly like. With any luck this will communicate itself to your partner, thus cancelling out any resentment he may feel.

Before you get angry about his annoying habits, try being inventive in stopping them. If necessary pretend to like something that you know he dislikes, then engineer a trade. Anger builds up tension and a combative atmosphere which you want to avoid just now.

Robert thought his designer stubble looked rakish. 'Yes,' agreed Jacqueline. 'It rakes my face and fanny.' He wouldn't shave it off. Jacqueline begged, glowered and threw tantrums. No success. In the end she found a beautiful cure for Robert's stubbornness: she stuck large pieces of elastoplast all over her chin and kept turning up at his office. Robert was embarrassed into surrender – and they actually ended up laughing about it.

All in all the most important thing with your various worries and grievances is beginning to examine them. It is very important that you don't embark on any of the exercises pretending that this time everything will suddenly be different.

PREPARING YOUR BODY: SOME OF THE TROUBLES

For the purposes of this programme 'preparing your body' is really another way of saying 'preparing your mind'. Because our attitude to our own bodies can be one of the most bothersome disruptions to our mental relaxation.

Feeling at ease with your own body is a keystone to sexual fulfilment. Nobody who is embarrassed about being seen nude, anxious about being overweight, or encumbered with uncomfortable garments is going to have an easy time.

Now I am aware that this is simple to say but very much more difficult to achieve. Let's face it, most women worry to an uncomfortable degree about what they look like. Even the most exquisite woman is very rarely flawless in her own eyes.

It is, of course, a cliché now to observe that from birth women are undermined about their bodies. We are constantly exhorted to be slender, alluring, fragrant, beautiful, sultry-lipped, wide-eyed – whatever the fashions of the day demand. Glossy magazines scream glamour and Page 3 girls give us all a complex by displaying flawless breasts every breakfast time. As one usually self-confident woman remarked: 'Just going to work on the tube each morning upsets me. There you are, surrounded by twenty editions of the "perfect girl" and you're uncomfortably conscious that the bloke you're going to strip off for this evening might also have been gazing at those oh-so-perfect breasts. Nice way to start the day, isn't it?'

The day I become prime minister the first new law I'll draw up is 'Page 3 Men' – so that a handsome hunk with a perfect body and huge, beautifully shaped penis stares at every man on the underground each morning. That would certainly be an effective way of showing male readers just how withering to a person's self-confidence this constant reminder of the currently 'desirable specimen' can be.

There are certain places where you expect perfect-looking women – *Vogue*, for example. But just to illustrate how all-pervasive this nonsense is, the drawing opposite is taken from a popular sex manual written by two long-standing and highly reputable American sex therapists – a manual currently recommended by Relate, the Marriage Guidance Council. And would you believe it, *on the facing page* the writers advise women to

> pay particular attention to where your standards are coming from . . . Chances are that your ideals have been adopted from television, magazines, and films in which the stereotypical woman is still *large breasted, slim, flawlessly complexioned, stylish, somewhat athletic, and barely twenty-three.* [My italics.] The image is as fictitious as an afternoon soap opera.

Feminists, of course, urge that we should not try to please men, but learn to live with ourselves. Very good advice, if only we could take it. But what is sound in theory is often very hard to do in practice.

You may be lucky and feel perfectly at ease with your own body. If not, *for this programme the important thing is that you strike a balance*. That is, a balance between coming to terms with what you consider your less pleasing features, and making an effort to change them. You must strive to feel as relaxed as you can about your own body, without getting into a tizzy about how to change it.

Self-help groups and assertiveness training can be encouraging. I found that the most helpful thing was exchange of views with other women. Knowing the kinds of problem they suffer, problems one very often never suspected, is a simple but effective counter to the 'perfection' of magazine images.

'O, THAT THIS TOO TOO SOLID FLESH WOULD MELT'

Shakespeare's lines were not, of course, meant literally. Hamlet, after all, had problems other than his figure (he's usually played by a skinny little actor, anyway). But they fit the facts here.

I grew up in the era of Twiggy and during those years never ceased to worry that I too was not a sylph. I remember how, because Twiggy and other models of the period were as flat as an ironing board, I used to try to squash my chest with tight clothes and, when that failed, I never went anywhere without clutching a large book to my chest. It makes me hoot with laughter now. God knows what the neighbours must have thought.

What a ludicrous situation! I wanted to be 'attractive' but I didn't have the knowledge or sophistication to realize that even if fashion dictates we all look like broomhandles, fashion rarely dictates men's sexual preferences (at least not from year to year). And I certainly didn't have the self-confidence to realize I could live without every man's approval anyway.

Like most other women, I've been on and off diets for years. Some work, some don't, some are sensible and some absurd. Now, whenever I begin a diet I think of Christina Rossetti's lines:

> Better by far you should forget and smile
> Than that you should remember and be sad

It's not just an admirable sentiment; it's an extremely useful dieting tip. The surest way to fail on a diet is to be constantly preoccupied with it. Dieters, because they want to lose weight quickly, cannot stop thinking about food. They're constantly mulling over what foods they're allowed, pining for those they're not, and every few hours jump on the scales hoping to see a difference. The outcome is – almost always – giving up. The results just aren't quick enough, and the continual concentration is exhausting.

So begin your diet, then 'forget and smile'. Don't let dieting preoccupy you. You *can't* change your shape in days, however manically you try. To see results will take weeks. Accept this fact. Draw up a list of your favourite dietary principles, the ones that suit you. That way you're far more likely to stick to them. Then forget.

IN THE BEDROOM

Exactly what you wear in bed and how you arrange your bedroom are, of course, personal matters and not my business. However, for the purposes of this plan, let me suggest the following general points:

1) *Don't* wear a lot of make-up in bed – a small part of you will

be worrying that it will smudge. Besides, the lights will probably be dim enough not to need it.

2) Dress carefully for bed. Wear something that you *know* you feel at ease in. New outfits – even nighties – can prove uncomfortable in all sorts of ways. Dress flatteringly, but don't be afraid to cover yourself up. A man's long shirt or pyjama top never fails to look attractive and is extremely comfortable. It covers you well if you feel you need that, but you can undo as many buttons as you choose, either at the beginning of the evening or as things hot up.

Don't get yourself done up like a sacrificial victim in the regulation black stockings and suspenders. Not only are they dreadfully uncomfortable, but you are shifting the emphasis on to *his* gratification. And that breaks one of the fundamental rules of my programme. Besides, *he* doesn't *need* any help to climax. The last thing you want is to encourage him to do it more quickly. It's your turn now.

3) An attractive, comfortable bedroom will help your confidence. As I've said before, and will say at least another dozen times, don't underestimate the importance of apparently peripheral things like this. If your bedroom doesn't look right or makes you feel ill at ease, then change it. Don't compromise. But arrange it *to please yourself*. Don't get black silk sheets and a leopard-skin rug because you've heard that Mata Hari was successful this way. The chances are you'll feel self-conscious rather than sexy (and so will he). Spend a week or two planning and arranging it exactly how you've always envisaged it. Don't agonize about the colour. If you don't like it as it is choose another – it's worth the price of a can of paint to set yourself at ease. Hang up the pictures you like, and revitalize it altogether. Never mind the rest of the house. Make your bedroom a room where *you* feel comfortable, not a boudoir designed to kill.

4) From the point of view of this programme, the most important aspect of your room is lighting. Make sure that you are comfortable with it and that it shows you up in the way you prefer. You should have a couple of table lamps, with 60- or even 40-watt bulbs – a dim, low-angled light with plenty of suggestive shadow

61

is just the thing. If you worry about your appearance then this simple arrangement of lighting will help to relax you. But remember: only make changes for *your* comfort. If you feel good as you are, don't fuss. Go on to the next section.

5) Most important of all, always try to arrange that your lovemaking takes place at your house, not his. (That is, of course, assuming you have a bedroom of your own.) You will feel more at ease in a room that is familiar. When you have to go to the bathroom you will feel relaxed walking down your own corridor, with your own things handy. To use a rather macho analogy – but a useful one – in sports matches the home team usually has the advantage.

CONTRACEPTION

It is vitally important to the success of your sex life that you are happy with your contraception. Anxiety about getting pregnant is one of the commonest reasons for failure of orgasm. In fact there are authentic cases where anxiety about getting pregnant was the *only* barrier to the woman's orgasm; as soon as she was really able to set her mind at rest, she found she could climax. I cannot overstress the importance of finding the method of contraception that is *comfortable and convenient* for you, and above all *safe*.

SUCCESSFUL SEX: A GOLDEN RULE

This is something that, if it's unusual in your relationship, you may find hard to do at first. It is worth every effort to put it into operation as soon as possible:

If he does something in bed that you don't like
say so at the beginning

For example, if his method of rubbing your clitoris is painful, *don't* be shy to tell him. I know it's awkward, but, believe me, it'll be a thousand per cent more awkward when he's been doing it like that for six months.

First, you don't want to have to endure it for six months, or until you know him well enough to mention it. It's no good for your nerves, and it's rotten for your progress during this programme.

Secondly, if you tell him straightaway then it's barely embarrassing at all, providing you say so kindly. And by setting up a situation of frankness, he may be relieved to feel that *he* can tell *you* that you're pinching his balls when you fondle them. Imagine that you'd been doing your special technique for six months, and then suddenly he tells you that all along it has been uncomfortable. The dreadful embarrassment! You might well feel that there are other things you've been doing wrong. Your whole confidence would be undermined. So for both your sakes: *tell each other at the beginning*.

Thirdly, it's wrong on principle. Start making little concessions and you'll undermine your sense of control. Having the courage to tell him means you're well on the way to greater self-control.

LEARNING TO SAY NO

Learning to say no to sex when you don't want it is really part and parcel of the section above. But because it is so important for a woman I have given it a section of its own.

Nobody has the right to demand sex off another person. It doesn't matter if they have been married for sixty years. Remember: if *he* didn't want it, he wouldn't *be able* to do it.

How you say no is important. Be pleasant, but firm. Don't get into the habit of making excuses such as 'headache' – you don't have to make excuses. It may seem simpler at first, but it's seriously undermining your stance in the relationship. If you really have a headache, then say, 'I have a headache.' If you are tired say 'I am tired.' Remember you are an *equal*, and you have the perfect right to say no if you feel no. By making excuses you are belittling yourself and your rights.

Also, it *is* hurtful to the man when he realizes (as he will sooner or later) that you are making excuses. It's hurtful because there is nothing he can grasp hold of – just an undermining sense of your dislike of sex, which is far more sinister and threatening than a truth that he can attempt to remedy. If you make a habit of being perfectly open, he has at least the opportunity to understand *why* you may not be feeling like it.

NO ORGASM: TO TELL OR NOT TO TELL?

A major issue facing women who do not climax at all is: 'Do I *tell* a new man that I've never had an orgasm?' As I have described at length in Chapter 2, this was a question I used to dread.

In general, my advice is don't mention it. As always, ultimately the details of your disclosure or secrecy will depend on you, your partner, and the relationship you have. If he is understanding and his concern about your lack of orgasm will help you, then by all means sit him down, begin with something like 'Nobody else has made me get so close,' and then spill the beans. But do it before you have sex, not during.

In the meantime, ensure that your sex life suits your requirements as much as possible. If you want more time during sex, remember that it is one of the standard fears of a man that he is too quick. Make use of this. After all, successful intercourse depends on mutual enjoyment – if it's not slow enough for you, then he hasn't met his side of the bargain.

In a long-term relationship the question 'Have you had an orgasm?' may well have cropped up already, and you will have your own way of dealing with it. It is really only a burning issue in a new relationship. I believe the best possible answer is to look critically at *him* and reply 'We'll see,' thus shifting the emphasis from your ability to his performance. Never look flustered or guilty.

Make it quite clear that the question is meaningless in the abstract like that – that the answer depends as much, if not a good deal more, on him as on you. Similarly, if, while you're in the middle of having sex, he asks 'Haven't you come yet?', with a nasty edge to his voice, give as good as you get – 'With *this* performance?' Shrug the blame off you and on to him. Always remember, sex is a two-way relationship.

Alternatively you can say, 'No, I've not yet had an orgasm, but don't let's get worked up about it.' Try to avoid making it an issue of great importance at this stage. This leaves you free to pursue your own training as freely as possible.

Or you can fake an orgasm. If you feel the need to do this, then you should familiarize yourself with Chapter 14.

THE SEXIEST DAYS OF YOUR LIFE?

Which part of the month do you feel most sexy?

Unlike other animals, women have the great advantage that they can mate and, a more dubious bonus, conceive all the year long. However, some days in the month you will feel sexier than others. And since in terms of sexual arousal we welcome all the help we can get, it's well worth noticing which days out of the twenty-eight you feel most sexy.

Shere Hite reports that most women who answered her questionnaire found that they noticed increased sexual desire before and during menstruation. Her conclusion, however, is the only incidence where I disagree with her. She says: 'Women are generally more interested in sex during times of the month when they are not fertile. This agrees with findings of other sex researchers.' To put it bluntly, sex researchers rarely agree about anything, and matters concerning the menstrual cycle are no exception. Whichever book you pick up seems to say something different, as a recent paper by two Canadians (Markowitz and Brender) confirms. Summarizing the research of the last few years, they note that some investigators have found the peak of erotic desire to be just after menstruation, others just before it. Others still suggest that it is around the time of ovulation; and some have found two or even three peaks. Then of course there are those who report no particular period of female sexual interest. (It's worth bearing in mind that while many women say they feel particularly sexy just after their period, this may be due to abstinence during their bleeding, and not to any special 'peak'.)

Here's an excellent opportunity for us to do our own research. Note that the double digit – 5.1 – refers to the chapter and to the exercise itself, for easy reference.

Exercise 5.1 Using Chart A on page 68, keep a record of your monthly cycle. Day 1 represents the first day of your period – and so on. All I want you to do is mark with a cross those days when you feel particularly sexy.

Don't start racking your brains each day to try and work out if you feel sexy or not. The chances are you won't be able to decide, and you'll end up confused. Forget about it overall, but on those days when you notice that you quite definitely *do* feel rather horny, then jot it down.

After a few weeks you may well find that you notice a pattern. If so, it's silly not to arrange to see your lover on those days. Of course if you live with your partner permanently, you may decide there is no advantage to knowing which days you are most likely to feel horny, since any time you do you can inveigle him into bed. But it's still worth doing the exercise, as any little piece of information about your own sexuality is helpful. You never know when it may come in useful in the future.

But more importantly, you may decide to introduce new exercises from the plan on those days that find you at your most responsive.

Naturally I am not suggesting that the thing works like clockwork. Many of you will find there is no pattern whatsoever, and this doesn't matter one bit. Besides, our attitude to sex is affected by all sorts of other factors: our personal state of mind, our relations that particular day with our partner, how we feel about our own body, even the weather. In olden times it was generally believed that desire peaks in the spring, when birds and animals are merrily breeding.

A friend of mine worked in the ticket office of a large opera company. A certain woman – large, red-headed, flamboyant – and her shy male escort used to visit the opera once a month. As they arrived, he always stood quietly nearby, while she went straight to the advance booking office and, after some preliminary counts on her fingers, requested two seats exactly twenty-eight days hence. Eventually this fell on a Sunday, when there was no performance. My friend, full of curiosity, enquired whether the date really needed to be so exact. 'Oh well, a day or two won't make much difference,' replied the lady, beaming, and then proceeded to explain that she was a married woman who lived in the country. On the pretence of staying overnight with a female friend, she visited the opera with her lover. 'And,' she concluded with a flourish, 'it's so much more successful if I see that it coincides with the *sauciest time of the month.*'

You may not be able to plot your 'sauciest time of the month' as accurately as she did, but like her the secret is to become familiar with yourself. Learn to recognize those moods and sensations that indicate you are ready for sex, not because *he* decides he wants it but because *your body is telling you*.

Chart A: your sexual desire

Day 1 represents the first day of your period. Mark X if you feel
noticeably sexy that day (regardless of whether you've actually
had sex or not). Compare your results over three months.

Exercise 5.2 Chart B is for recording your responsiveness on
days when you have had sex. The idea is to evaluate your degree
of arousal. For example, if on Day 1 you feel highly aroused, mark
the appropriate level on the chart. Once you have gathered some
data you can compare your findings with Chart A.

Chart B: your sexual responsiveness

For every day that you have sex mark a dot against one of the following levels on how you enjoyed the experience. If you achieve orgasm encircle the dot.

Did not enjoy it
Medium quality
Good quality

SUPERTIP

Have you ever wished you could make love during your menstrual period, without all the mess? You can! Ask your doctor to fit you with a diaphragm contraceptive device. If this is not your usual form of contraception you may have to pay for it, but it's well worth the money. Whenever you want to have sex during your period, just put it in – not, of course, as a contraceptive (you *must* use your usual method as well) but simply to stop the blood.

If your flow is particularly heavy, you may notice a little staining on the sheet, but nothing more. But take care when you remove the diaphragm afterwards – do so over the lavatory, or squatting in the bathtub – because the blood collects in the hollow.

KEGEL EXERCISES

It has long been known that a well-toned vagina greatly increases the pleasure of the male, as the following somewhat over-the-top description of one woman's 'nutcracker' technique, taken from a nineteenth-century French work *Tableaux Vivants*, makes clear:

> I entered, I thrust – Ai'e! Heaven! What pleasure! The coynte of this chambermaid was like a rasp! This waiting-maid had that which Duchesses had not, that which I had vainly sought in Marquises – the CASSE-NOISETTE. It tightened on me, it pinched me. And these pinches and this vice, acting as a furious suction pump on my surprised member, astonished me. I enjoyed, I discharged, I sank with all my weight . . .

The really good news, however, is that *women* also benefit.

In 1952 Dr Arnold Kegel developed a series of exercises for women who needed to improve urinary control by strengthening the pubococcygeal or P-C muscle, which controls the size and tension of the vaginal opening. Much to his patients' delight, it turned out that the exercises increased their ability to have orgasms; it also increased the intensity of them. By building up the strength of the muscle, they had increased the blood flow to it, and since good blood flow plays a very important part in sexual arousal the result was greater sexual sensitivity and responsiveness.

Kegel exercises are not as popular as they once were, but some sex therapists still recommend them. I am convinced they work, and that good muscle tone in the right place really does help orgasm. By carrying out some simple exercises you can significantly increase the quality and the quantity of your orgasms. So if you don't have a well exercised P-C then start working out.

First of all you've got to make sure you know which muscle I'm talking about. The way to do this is by interrupting your urine flow when you go to the toilet – the muscle you use to control the flow is the P-C muscle. Make sure you've got the right muscle by checking that your control doesn't depend on your legs being close together. You don't want to build up big thigh muscles by accident!

Once you feel you've got a hold on the P-C then start exercising it. The wonderful thing is that you can do these exercises at any time, in the middle of the supermarket or in the privacy of your own bedroom, standing, sitting or lying. Like other exercises, they'll be a little tiring to do at first but they'll quickly become much easier.

Exercise 5.3

1. Contract and relax the muscle. Do this twenty times.
2. Contract the muscle, hold for three seconds, and then relax. Do this ten times.
3. Contract the muscle while inhaling. Try to avoid contracting your stomach muscle at the same time. This will be difficult at first, but it becomes easier with practice. Do this ten times.

That's it. Do them three to four times a day. For both you and your partner it'll be well worth the effort.

THE QUESTIONNAIRE

Pick up a pen and a piece of paper. In just a moment I want you to answer a very personal questionnaire.

It is important that you answer carefully and in detail. If necessary, illustrate your replies with stories and anecdotes, even drawings. But, most important of all, you must answer with complete honesty. This is not always easy to do with such a sensitive matter as sex, let alone orgasm. So if you're sitting in a public place turn over to a later section and come back to this one only when you're well and truly on your own. If you're with someone else who's insisting that you go ahead with it right now, then go ahead, and lie your soul away whenever necessary. But return to the questionnaire later, when alone, and tell the truth. It is important, for the success of this programme, that you are fully aware of your own strengths and weaknesses.

Answer the questions in whatever order you like. Once you've finished you can burn them, turn them into paper aeroplanes or lock them up in a secret drawer.

Best of all, send them to me care of the publisher. This will serve two functions. On the one hand, if you're anything like me, knowing someone else wants to see them will make you answer the questions more fully and carefully. On the other hand, your answers will provide unique and fascinating material for a broad-ranging, international survey of women, sex and orgasm, the like of which has never been done before. Of course your answers will be treated in strictest confidence – in fact, you needn't send your name at all. And you can fictionalize the irrelevant, non-sexual details if you feel the need.

Enough of this delay. Get ready with your pen. Let yourself go!

INTRODUCTORY

1. Does the word orgasm embarrass you? Why?

2. Does the thought of other people knowing you have this book embarrass you? Which people and why?

3. Do you think orgasms are overrated?

MASTURBATION

4. How often do you masturbate? Does the frequency with which you masturbate vary? If never, why not?

5. Do you find masturbation enjoyable both physically and psychologically?

6. Do you have an orgasm every time you masturbate? Usually? Sometimes? Rarely? Give details.

7. What is the greatest number of orgasms you've had during one masturbation 'session'? Do they vary in intensity? On the whole how many do you need to feel really satisfied?

INTERCOURSE

8. How often (roughly speaking) do you have an orgasm during intercourse? Never? Rarely? Sometimes? Usually? Always? Think about this carefully. Don't over-estimate: Remember, when I began, my reply to this would have been a solemn 'never'.

9. If never, do you feel that you have ever come close? Do you know what prevented you from getting there?

10. Have you ever felt desperate because there seemed to be *no reason* why you shouldn't have an orgasm?

11. Is it easier for you to have an orgasm during intercourse if you stimulate the clitoral area directly with your hand at the same time? Can you have an orgasm without added clitoral stimulation?

12. Do you ever feel physical discomfort during intercourse? Do you know why?

ORAL/MANUAL

13. Do you enjoy manual sex physically and psychologically?

14. Do you enjoy oral sex physically and psychologically?

15. Do you find it easy to have orgasms during manual sex? If not, why not?

16. Do you find it easy to have orgasms during oral sex? If not, why not?

SEX IN GENERAL

17. Does the quality of your orgasm depend on what type of sex you have? How does orgasm from masturbation compare with orgasm from sex with your partner?

18. Do your orgasms vary in intensity? If so, can you think of any circumstances which influence the intensity?

19. Does the time of the month make any difference to your enjoyment of sex?

20. Are there any times when you don't mind about not having an orgasm, even if your partner does have one? When you do mind, how strongly do you mind?

21. Do you think your difficulty with orgasm affects your attitude to sex? Does it affect (in so far as you can tell) your attitude to men? To life in general?

22. Have you ever felt when you were unable to have an orgasm during sex that it was your 'fault'? Why? Has your lover ever implied that it was your 'fault'?

23. In your opinion is it true that most women are less interested in sex than men? How about orgasm?

24. Do you think men dislike women who initiate sex? Should a woman be submissive during sex?

25. Do you think that women are more emotional about sex than men? How would you compare the average woman's sex drive with the average man's?

26. Are fantasies important to you during sex? What sort of fantasies?

27. Have you ever had an orgasm during your sleep, i.e. a nocturnal orgasm.

28. Do you ever feel self-conscious during sex? Why?

29. If you and your partner like different things during sex, how often do you have it your way?

30. Do you fake orgasms frequently? Sometimes? Rarely? Never? If you have ever faked your orgasm, why did you do it? If not, why not?

31. How easy do you think it is for your partner to tell if you've had a genuine orgasm or not? How easy do you think it would be for a person you'd only been to bed with once to tell?

32. Do you ever feel intimidated by the constant media preoccupation with sex? For example, that you may not be as sexually sophisticated or as skilled as other women?

33. Sex manuals often talk of sex and orgasm as profoundly beautiful and significant, one of the greatest experiences life has to offer. Do you ever feel that your experiences cannot match up to this ideal?

34. On the whole how useful have you found sex manuals to your lovemaking? Have you learned more from them than, say, talking to friends? When I say 'learned' I mean learned things that you *enjoy*, not simply what you are 'supposed' to enjoy.

35. Is there anything else you would like to add? Do you have any tips, however odd or silly, for women who have difficulty with orgasm? Any stories that are revealing or helpful?

CHAPTER SIX

STEP 1:
THE MIRROR

This programme began the moment you picked up the book. The early chapters, apart from giving you information about myself and our – womankind's – difficulties with orgasm, were written to help you realize that you are not alone, and that there is an enormous amount you can do for yourself. You've already been asked to answer a questionnaire and write down your worries, fears, disappointments and hopes for the future. You are starting to treat your difficulty with professionalism and determination. You are already on the path to success.

Now you have finished the introductory part of this programme, it is time to start training and begin the plan.

I have stressed the importance of feeling at ease with your own body. As this ease develops, so will your sense of relaxation about orgasm and your self-confidence.

So, let's begin with a splash. Light-heartedly.

Take an evening off alone, when you know you will not be disturbed. You must have at least two hours for this, preferably more. Disconnect the telephone and pour yourself a drink. Choose some music that really gives you pleasure. It might be gentle, soothing classical music. It might be a romantic love song. Or it might be a jazzy, exhilarating disco tune.

Now rig up a good-sized mirror. It needn't be a full-length one, but can be a wall mirror, a bathroom mirror or whatever – just so long as you have a good view of your face and at least half, preferably all, of your body.

You will also need good lighting: not strong, uncompromising bulbs, but flattering, angled lighting, such as a photographer uses to get the best from his shots – after all, that's exactly how models get to look as good as they do in the pictures. If necessary borrow some lamps from another room. Don't stint and compromise. If the lights still aren't right, buy a pink bulb or two.

Now you are going to fix your face, hair and body exactly how you like it. Begin with a long, relaxing, scented bath. Then sit down and make yourself look as delicious as you like. By that I do not mean how you would make yourself look if you were going out to an important dinner party. I mean how you – in all your dreams – would like yourself to look, regardless of other people. (I first used this step after I'd broken up with a man who'd been particularly unpleasant in our parting argument. I went home, poured myself a strong cocktail, and flattered myself until I fell asleep.) Your ideal 'look' may be sweet, demure and romantic, or it may be outrageous and bold. Susan, for humorous example, has always had a secret longing to dress up as a barmaid in a Wild West film:

> You know, one of those really curvy women who heaved their chests up into a basque. I bought one but I've never dared wear it. One night I put it on, along with some fish-net tights. I noticed the tights had a great rip in them – then I thought, no, that's all part of it. I bunched together a load of petticoats and put on some high heels. I thought I looked great and was prancing around the flat having a merry time. I ended up quite drunk as well – well, a *barmaid*, I *had* to . . . I wish I'd had a photographer there. I'd never have done that except in private. The next week my best friend and I did it together. It was the best evening of the year.

Annie dresses in black.

Step 1: The Mirror

**All black. Then I powder my face so that it's ashen. It's
really startling. I wish I had the nerve to go out like that.**

In short, you are going to play at being what you fantasize
about being. If you want to pose as a scantily clad model, then go
right ahead: to hell with your principled objections to girlie
magazines – this is not for the titillation of some anonymous man,
this is for *yourself*. Sometimes I like wearing high-heeled leather
boots, and a long, deep-blue velvet cloak that I bought a few years
ago at an antique clothes market in London, with a silver-topped
cane and nothing else, and I imagine I'm going through the
dockyards late at night watched by hungry dockers who haven't
the nerve to approach. As I look at myself in the mirror I try and
give my stride just enough length to reveal my thigh.

Another friend of mine, an earnest socialist who does admirable
things like make her own sesame seed bread and pick mushrooms
in the autumn, pictures herself as a scandalous fur-clad social*ite*
with silk stockings and elegant smoking habits. She likes to talk
out loud and dazzle the imaginary company. Once people open up
about themselves, you learn the most curious secrets!

Roberta, who is distinctly large, explains that she likes

**to come home, and just pose without trying to cover up.
It's there that I can feel at ease with my size and don't
have to be continually seeing magazines advertising the
latest diet and all that nonsense. I like to stand with my
shawl around my waist, like one of those lovely island
women you see in their reed skirts. They're always pretty
ample, and not ashamed of it. I say to myself: 'Bobby, this
is what you've got. There's a lot of it, and you couldn't do
with an inch less!'**

Use whatever accessories you like – sexy panties, a shirt
revealingly draped. Put on high heels to make your legs look
alluring. You can pout, look over your shoulder, pose on a chair

the way the *Playboy* models do – it's all for your own immodest satisfaction!

As you look in the mirror, don't think: 'My God, I look sexy, I bet Harry/Sam/Steve or whoever would go for me.' Instead you must make the fine mental adjustment to 'God, I look good, full stop.' Gently shift your emphasis *away* from pleasing the man *towards* pleasing yourself.

As you stand there in front of the mirror, remove a garment or two. Let the shawl slip from your shoulders. Unhook a suspender and roll your stocking top down. Undo the buttons on the front of your blouse. Gradually, little by little, reveal your body. Reveal it so that at all stages it pleases you.

I want you simply to enjoy watching yourself and your body in the mirror. Instead of your usual critical examination standing on the scales, pinching the inches here and there, and groaning about the cellulite on your hips, you are going to *pose* in the most alluring way you can. You need not remove all your clothes. Take off as many pieces as you feel comfortable with. Turn round and look at yourself from behind, over your own shoulder, with perhaps your shirt hitched up over one buttock. If you don't like the shape of your breasts pose in such a way that they do please you.

While you are doing this, try taking a little body oil and rubbing it over yourself. You may or may not take to this: some women hate it (I'm one of them), but others find it a wonderful feeling, smoothing it over their breasts and the curve of their thighs.

If you have a camera with delayed action shutter release (not at all uncommon nowadays, even on inexpensive cameras) take some photos of yourself. If not, simply try pointing the camera at the mirror. You won't get your face (because of the flash) but you'll probably get the rest of you. Best of all, do this exercise with a close friend and take photos of each other. If you feel nervous about what the chemist might think, use a Polaroid. Once developed, take out any you hate, get hold of a pair of vicious-looking scissors and ritually *snip them to pieces*. Keep the rest where you can continue to look at them. They'll do wonders for your confidence.

The idea is simply to see yourself in the most flattering and attractive angle, and as somebody with *power* – the power to please yourself, to get what you want out of sex. It is no more than a frivolous exercise; but it is also the first step in gaining control over your own body.

And that's it.

Once you have indulged in your first celebration (it's most important that you don't neglect it) you are ready to progress to step 2. Repeat this simple, undemanding, rather theatrical exercise whenever you want to.

CHAPTER SEVEN

STEP 2: MASTURBATION

The foundation stone of your sexual progress is learning to achieve orgasm on your own. It is the easiest part, and it is also extremely pleasurable.

Masturbation is important to my programme for two reasons:

(1) It trains your body to respond sexually. For obvious reasons, this is best done when you are alone and at your most relaxed. Once you have learned what your *basic* sexual needs are, and how best to satisfy them, then you will be a long way towards your goal. You will then progress to experimenting with masturbation, learning a variety of ways of coming to orgasm in private. This is absolutely crucial, because

(2) Masturbation is a means of self-control, of exercising control over your own body. As I have already pointed out, control is a vital factor in your sexual fulfilment. By thoroughly familiarizing yourself with your own sexuality, and experimenting with it, you learn government over it. At the end of this stage of the programme you will be able to masturbate successfully in many different ways. This is a skill you must acquire. It takes time and patience, but once acquired it will never leave you. You will be ready to continue your training in intercourse.

It is also worth noting that almost all professional sex researchers and therapists recognize masturbation as a vital path to achieving orgasm during sex.

ABOUT MASTURBATION

Virtually all women who masturbate can do so to orgasm. Think about that: it's an amazing fact. Women who have never managed to have an orgasm with a partner can almost always have one on their own quite happily and quickly.

Even so, ignorance and guilt are *still* obstacles preventing women from masturbating. Ignorance is comparatively easy to overcome. Just read on! Guilt is more difficult. So for the sake of those who find masturbation shameful, I want to spend a little time discussing the subject. I don't expect to help you overcome your feelings in so brief a space – from bitter experience I know that these feelings can run deep. I also know how infuriating it is when someone tries to solve your difficulties with a few trite phrases. But, as one who has herself experienced great inhibitions with masturbation, I do hope that I can help you to overcome those obstacles – by dint of patience, encouragement and practice – showing that you too can learn as I have done.

Some women begin masturbating when they are children without even knowing what it is they are doing. Many stumble upon it later, by accident: they feel an urge between their legs, begin to rub themselves, and then, rather unexpectedly, reach orgasm.

My friend Laurelle discovered masturbation because she loved jigsaw puzzles:

> Several years ago I was living in a poky little place in Edinburgh. I didn't have much money then and instead of going out in the evening I used to spend most of the time drowning my sorrows with 5000-piece puzzles. None of the tables were big enough so I had to spread them out on the floor in front of the fire. Since I always sat with my legs bent underneath, the heel of my foot pressed between my legs, and as I reached out to get the piece I wanted – well, all I can say is that things started looking up a bit. It used to give me a real thrill to do it when

**a friend came round, especially one of my flatmate's
numerous boyfriends!**

Funnily enough, I recently came across a very similar method
of masturbation, in Sai Kaku's *Life of an Amorous Woman*, but this
time practised several hundred years ago in Japan.

**One day, as I was examining a fascinating depiction by
Hishikawa of an erotic scene, I was stirred despite myself
to the most intense excitement. I sought then to quench my
amorous flames, now with my heel, now the middle finger
of my hand. These were cold and insensible tools indeed
for stilling my wanton lust, and soon I was overcome with
desire for a more solid form of love.**

Personally, I was quite old when I began masturbating – well
into my twenties. I had never tried it, never wanted to try it, and
hardly knew what it involved. I remember that around this time
there was a great deal of fuss in the newspapers over a very
advanced new sex education film which showed a young woman –
a schoolteacher apparently – masturbating. I thought I knew the
meaning of the word 'masturbation', yet I had literally no idea
what this woman could be doing to herself. The possibility of
orgasm never entered my head. As I never saw the film, it was still
a while before I found out. Sitting in a tree watching an extremely
dull cricket match, I discovered with a rush of pleasure what all
the publicity was about.

For several weeks after I made my discovery, I would make any
excuse to go to bed early so as to enjoy myself. But every time I
felt a pang of guilt. I worried that I was doing something wrong;
not so much that it was wrong in the eyes of God – it was always
my opinion that he would be little interested in my physical
weaknesses, and concern himself more with my spiritual failings –
but that it was wrong in the eyes of society and nature. It was such
an intimate, self-centred sort of pleasure – all that concentration
on your own satisfaction indicates something unseemly, rather like
an obese glutton sitting alone with platefuls of caviare, Turkish

delight and vintage wine, and not sharing it with anybody. It had to be done in private, on the sly. I was constantly worried that someone would knock on the door, or peek through the curtains, or hear me breathing.

People rarely discuss masturbation openly and honestly. At best, the common reaction is giggling, sniggering and blushing. At worst the very word has a nasty ring to it – it not only sounds unpleasant, but actually derives from the Latin *manu-stuprare* meaning 'to defile with the hand'. Added to which the slang term for a person who masturbates – wanker – is a particularly scathing term of abuse.

I know that when I walked down the street just after I had indulged, I felt that my guilt was written large all over me. If I happened to catch the eye of a passer-by, I'd blush with shame, feeling like Mary McCarthy's heroine Libby in *The Group* who

> had a little secret; she sometimes made love to herself, on the bath mat, after having her tub. She always felt awful afterwards, sort of shaken and depleted and wondering what people would think if they could see her, especially when she took herself what she called 'Over the Top'.

After a while I forced myself to give it up. My word, what agony that was! I felt noble – occasionally. But then as soon as I began to dwell on my new-found virtue, the desire sprang up afresh.

We all know that sex talk can be embarrassing. But it puzzled me why masturbation should be a doubly shameful thing. After all, not only is it enjoyable but it costs nothing, it harms nobody, and it is *safe*. Because we do not risk venereal disease from a partner, it should be viewed as a particularly *clean* form of pleasure, yet the atmosphere that surrounds it is one of murky nastiness.

Actually, I reckon it's a lot to do with men. After all, when men masturbate they discharge semen. During sex with a partner, the semen is neatly 'contained'. In masturbation the wet, sticky mess is liable to spill in the most awkward places. No wonder masturbation is deemed 'dirty'.

Of course here women have a great advantage over men: no mess, nothing to show. I've often roared with laughter over my friend Sam's tales of the difficulties that men have in relieving themselves.

> Sometimes you simply have to do it, like it or not. But believe me, it can be misery. First of all an erection is no easy thing to conceal – it's terribly embarrassing when you're just stepping on to a crowded tube and bang, for no reason in particular, you get a bloody great hard-on. There you are standing with your whatsit on a level with all those seated passengers, desperately trying to keep your newspaper in place. And there's no possibility of relieving yourself unobtrusively. In this respect at least I really envy women.

Masturbation still carries overtones of guilt and selfishness, maybe even pathos. In Victorian times masturbation was considered the cause of everything from nose-bleeds to insanity. Early this century the US Patent Office even granted a patent for a masturbation alarm that rang in the parents' bedroom when the child's bed began moving in a suggestive way! And did you know that in 1898 an anti-masturbatory food was invented which was supposed to take away all sexual desire – Corn Flakes.

Religion also tends to have a bad effect on women's tendency to masturbate, but despite what the vicar might say, modern biblical scholars accept that there is no criticism of masturbation anywhere in the Bible. And what references there are, are to male masturbation, anyway. The real condemnation in the Bible is not of masturbation, but of wasting semen that might have been (on certain occasions) put to better use. Onan, for example, was killed by the Lord because 'he spilled it on the ground' instead of impregnating his brother's wife Tamar, as God expected him to do. In short, he was condemned for practising *coitus interruptus*, a primitive form of contraception. The fact that 'onanism' is used today to mean 'masturbation' merely reflects the biblical ignorance of the person who coined the term in the eighteenth century, rather than any disapproval on God's part.

For about fifteen years, since I sat watching the cricket match that fateful day, I felt ashamed of private sex. It was only in my early thirties that I started to feel the self-confidence to think the matter over slowly and analytically. *The Hite Report on Female Sexuality* was perhaps the greatest liberation. Here at last was a forum in which not just a few, but thousands of women were talking about subjects with complete honesty, free of the usual mockery and guilt. I was not, I discovered, in the least bit unusual in my private sexual needs, neither was I alone in having difficulty coming to terms with them. Over 80 per cent of women in *Hite* admitted to masturbating, and the figure is even higher for men. Another person's expression of worries and reactions similar to one's own can have a very therapeutic effect. Furthermore, masturbation is extremely good for you. *A woman's ability to have an orgasm during masturbation is widely regarded as one of the best ways of determining her sexual potential*. It is an indication of natural desires and sexual behaviour; it is one of the ways in which your body learns about its sexuality and comes to terms with it; it is also one of the ways your body relieves itself of sexual tension that would otherwise have to find some less pleasant outlet. Finally, as sexologists agree, it is a simple and highly effective means to help you to become fully orgasmic.

You'd be surprised how many times masturbation crops up in literature. The heroine in *The Story of O*

> remembered seeing her friend Marion doing it. O had been only fifteen years old. Marion had sat in an armchair in a hotel room, with one leg flung over an arm and her head sagging to the other, caressing herself and moaning in front of O. She had once done it in her office and her boss had come in and caught her . . .

I remember one day in the library picking up a book that showed an old-fashioned advertisement for some complicated patent gadgetry involving leather straps and metal clasps designed to be worn at night by Victorian males to prevent nocturnal erections, masturbation and wet dreams. Well, I thought, what in the world can be more *un*natural than that? I laughed out loud and suddenly felt a whole lot better.

Then I began to realize that animals do it; even out in the open. Standing around the primate cages (our distant ancestors, remember) at London Zoo was an enlightening experience. I got so interested I even looked it up in the library. In one of the books that I finally summoned the courage to order from the request stacks, I read that

> **Female mammals in peak heat may resort to rubbing their sensitive genitalia rythmically on the ground or on sharp projections, thus creating the stimulus of a penis jerking in and out. Female cats regularly resort to this kind of simulated intercourse. Female monkeys do it by tweaking their clitoris. Female talapoin monkeys finger themselves through their back legs, becoming more and more excited.**
>
> (J. Sparks, *The Sexual Connection*)

That same book goes on to talk about a bottle-nosed dolphin who lived off the south-west coast of England, who used to sidle up to boats, 'his massive pink penis rubbing against the hull'. Once again, what could I do but hoot with laughter? Always a very liberating response.

Picking up some anthropology books I learned that many tribes regard both male and female masturbation as vital to an individual's development. Amongst the Bala peoples of Africa, little girls masturbate first with their fingers and later with something called a 'kankondenkonde' – a dildo made of manioc root.

More and more I became convinced that masturbation was a perfectly ordinary function, that virtually everybody does it, and that many more would happily do it if our culture weren't still emerging from the repressive sexual atmosphere of the last century. And this is certainly the view endorsed by almost every medic and therapist in the West. As for the East, they've known about these things far longer than we have. As one doctor friend told me, the only way that masturbation can be construed as harmful is when it causes guilt.

Now, whenever I think of masturbation, instead of imagining something sordid and greedy, I visualize those wonderful masterpieces by Goya: *Maya Clothed* and *Maya Naked*, or Titian's nudes, that really put one in the mood.

Unfortunately there are still some women who cannot get rid of superstitions. They worry that having an orgasm alone means they will be less able to do so with a man. Others find it depressing, lonely, empty, dirty, cheap.

That's old-fashioned talk. But if you cannot rid yourself of it, think of it this way. In this programme masturbation is nothing more than a means to an end. Quite apart from being a perfectly innocent, safe and satisfying pleasure, it's the route by which women can learn how to make the most of sex. Masturbation is the means to satisfying lovemaking with a partner – and when I say satisfying I mean satisfying for *both* of you. And, what's more, it's a great cure for insomnia.

HOW DO I MASTURBATE?

Of course, many of you will have been masturbating successfully for years and will have your own special method. You can skip this section and go to the next, on 'Improving Your Ability to Masturbate'. Do *not* skip that section, however. It is pivotal to your success with this programme.

For those who have never tried masturbation, let me suggest the following.

Complete relaxation is essential. Make sure you will not be disturbed. Disconnect the phone, close the curtains, shut the doors – do whatever is necessary to put yourself at ease and make you confident that you won't be interrupted. Since this is your first time, allow yourself at least an hour during which you know you can be alone. Some women climax very quickly; most women I've met who masturbate often can do so in under five minutes, although they might continue again and again for a long time after. But when you are beginning it is a good idea to allow yourself leeway; it helps you increase your relaxation, and you will probably find that like any other skills it takes a lot more concentration and effort to begin with than it will later on.

Put yourself to bed – alone, of course – and lie in a warm and comfortable position. If the thought of removing all your clothes makes you nervous, then leave some on. Above all, the most important thing is that you feel as at ease as possible.

Open your legs. Begin by exploring your body very gently with your hands, up and down your torso, over your breasts, in whichever way feels most enjoyable. Now bring your hands down between your legs. Gently explore all around the area of your genitals, probing and rubbing, in whichever manner pleases you most. You will probably find that one area is more sensitive than another and by using your fingers to manipulate it you can produce a pleasant sensation that seems to extend vaguely into other parts of your body. It is not the same as the pleasurable relief one derives from rubbing or scratching some other part of your body; it is warmer, making you slightly breathless and perhaps want to tense your legs, and it is much more directly *pleasurable*. But don't worry. You'll know it when you feel it. It is quite unlike any other sensation. The more you play with your hands in that area, the more the sensation will increase. This sensation is not an orgasm, but it is the run-up to one. If you keep it up, sooner or later the orgasm will follow: a sudden, intense climax of the sensations that preceded. Some of you will climax in five or ten minutes; others – especially to begin with – may well have to work at it for twenty or thirty. You may have to try it for days or even weeks, but providing you relax and do exactly what pleases you, you will succeed.

Your own hands are the most useful tool for masturbation: they are warm as well as uniquely sensitive. However, many women find that pressure from another object also produces satisfying sensations. When Nora began masturbating she used to use a rolled up sock which she pressed against herself. Susan always uses the arm of her teddy bear, which is soft and firm. The ways and circumstances in which women masturbate are legion. Some prefer a full and slow fantasy lasting an hour or more, others get straight to the point. Some get completely dressed up for the occasion, some look in the mirror while they do it, or rub their breasts. One woman I know stands in front of the mirror dressed only in a shirt and tie, and places a vibrator sticking out between her thighs, like an erect male member. Then by rubbing the vibrator she pretends to be a man masturbating. This gets her so worked up that she is able to climax almost without doing anything further. Another friend does it with her husband lying asleep beside her: 'Don't laugh,' she told me, 'but I learned to keep in rhythm with his snores, so that he wouldn't wake up.'

Perhaps the most dramatic masturbation scene is related in a French work of literature *L'Escole des Filles*, the story of

> a king's daughter who had made for her a bronze statue of a man, painted flesh colour, and furnished with a phallus of a more yielding material. This machine was erect and hollow, it had a red head and a small hole at the end, with two pendants in the shape of testicles, everything in close imitation of nature. When the damsel was inflamed by the presence of this figure, she approached the phallus and thrust it into her vulva, clasping the buttocks of the statue and drawing herself against it. When she was on the point of discharging she touched a certain spring which projected from the buttocks and the statue immediately squirted a warm and thickened liquor, white like pap, into the lady's vulva, thus satisfying her venereal desires.

Fur and feathers rubbed against breasts and inner thighs is another popular method, or sitting in a bathtub and directing the shower jet between the legs – even if it doesn't specifically lead to orgasm it's useful preparation. Other women do active movements against things, for example putting a pillow between their legs, or beneath them when lying down and using the effect of friction and pressure to lead them to climax. Some simply squeeze their thighs together. Most do a combination of things, depending on the circumstance and the degree of their desire. But the traditional way, with legs apart lying on the bed, seems to be the most popular – at least for novices.

Comparatively few women insert things into their vaginas. This is for a straightforward reason: the pleasure centre, the clitoris, is outside the vagina. Penetration into the vagina is not the primary stimulus to orgasm, although it may well serve to exaggerate the response induced through clitoral stimulation. I personally find the knowledge of there being a penis-like object within oneself very arousing. Ginny has a special method:

> I prefer to do it in the usual way, that is, lying down with my own hands. But just as I feel I'm about to climax I push a vibrator into me. Having something to contract around is far more satisfying than doing it with an empty vagina. I used to need to do it three or four times before I was satisfied, but this way just the once is enough.

Finding a suitable object to insert is not easy. Try looking for one and you'll begin to realize that the penis is really rather a well-designed object: it's not simply the shape, but the unique combination of firm yet soft, and warm as well. Objects that are too hard – like a hairbrush handle – are at best unsatisfying, and often painful. Carrots are clammy as well. Once, when I was in a hotel room in Bali, the waiter knocked on the door with a dish of exotic fruit. Feeling horny I sized up the man – and decided his bananas looked more appetizing than he did. When he'd shut the door I unpeeled this not-too-ripe banana and used it to great effect. This, I later discovered, was a favourite with the harem ladies of the Orient, who rarely had sufficient access to a man to satisfy their needs, and therefore had to be inventive with bulbs, roots and fruits – sometimes even with well-endowed statues.

While we're on the subject of artificial penises, some of you may decide to invest in a vibrator. They certainly have their uses, as Jessica found out:

> They're the right size and shape – a lot better than most other things I can think of – but even so they're not perfect. A bit too hard and unyielding. After all, they're

little more than a jazzed up stick of plastic. I tend to buy a smallish size – for some reason a vibrator always seems much larger and more 'filling' than a real cock, so a big one can be uncomfortable.

My own vibrator had an in-and-out thrusting movement which was pleasant. But buy a good quality one: mine broke because the contractions from my orgasm proved too strong for the motor, and it seized up! If you are using a vibrator, try unrolling a condom over it. This means the shaft slips into you more easily, and it creates a more realistic feel. If you don't go for that rather crude rubbery smell, try hunting out the new fruit-flavoured condoms.

Nuns are traditionally supposed to use altar candles, although Apollinaire describes an episode with a young boy who hears his aunt confessing to a priest the following story:

'Once my sister said to me, "Our maid uses up an awful lot of candles. She's obviously reading novels in bed, and one of these nights she'll end up setting the house on fire. You sleep near her, so you be careful!" That very evening, when I saw a light in the maid's room, here's what I did. I left the door open and tip-toed noiselessly into Kate's room. She was sitting on the floor with her back half-turned to me, and leaning towards her bed. In front of her was a chair with a mirror on it, and to the left and right of the mirror two candles were burning. Kate was in a nightgown and I distinctly observed in the mirror that she was holding something long and white and was manipulating this with both hands back and forth between her thighs, which were wide apart. She was sighing deeply and trembling all over. Suddenly I heard her cry: "Oh, oh, aah! it feels so good!" . . . She explained to me she was doing it in memory of her lover who had been conscripted into the army . . . I left, but the spectacle had left such a mark on me that afterwards, Father, I couldn't help trying the same thing, and alas! I've often repeated it since.'

Another important factor in masturbation is fantasy. So important, in fact, that I devote a whole chapter to it later on. Suffice to say here that working out your own particular fantasy can greatly stimulate your enjoyment.

IMPROVING YOUR ABILITY TO MASTURBATE

I have stressed that learning to masturbate is extremely important for this plan. Learning to masturbate *with ease and flexibility* is the real clue to success. You must become extremely accomplished at masturbation; only then are you beginning to acquire control over your own sexual responses. Until you are a real *expert* at seeing to your own pleasure you cannot be sure of having it with another person. Versatility is the keyword.

You are now at the stage where you are able to masturbate fairly easily. Having got this far in the programme I want to make an analogy. Think of yourself as the woman who has begun to learn a foreign language – Italian, for example. You have arrived in Naples, and after all your hours of perseverance with the Teach Yourself manual, you have mastered some phrases and expressions. You can manage basic things like ordering a meal in a restaurant or buying a ticket for the theatre – providing people speak slowly. You have broken the ice, but now you must learn fluency – even when people speak at their normal speed, without the helpful gestures.

So it is with your sexual training. Like the language student, you must learn *fluency*. That is, you must learn to bring yourself to orgasm in a variety of situations. As the course progresses you will see the wisdom of this advice more and more.

Those of you who have just begun to masturbate, will, as I said above, probably find that to succeed requires concentration and effort. You must simply press on, masturbating regularly whenever you have the desire and opportunity. I have no hesitation in saying that you will find your ability improves quickly – provided, of course, you are uninterrupted and in comfortable circumstances.

If you feel uneasy or guilty about devoting so much attention to your private sexual satisfaction, just remember that this is all part of a process; *it is a means to an end*. The end is to learn how to make your sex life with your partner more enjoyable *for both of you*.

How do I build up my skills?

There are two ways in which you build up your masturbation skills:

1) by gradually doing it more frequently,

2) by doing it in a variety of different situations. This creates the sexual *versatility* that is so important to your progress.

To begin with you will most likely find that after having achieved orgasm it will be some time before you are ready to do it again. Gradually, as you develop, you will be able to do it more frequently, with less effort. When I first began I could manage at best one orgasm a night, if I was lucky and if I concentrated hard. I'd masturbate as I settled down with a book. After a while I found that, with a half-hour break in between, I was ready for another go to send me off to sleep. Now I am versatile enough to masturbate in virtually any position, several times in a row. Likewise with the *circumstances* of your masturbation: to begin with you will need 'ideal conditions'. Gradually, like the language student, you will grow accomplished in ways that were previously quite impossible.

Below, I outline fifteen different ways of masturbating that you can practise. In each case, it is not sufficient to do it just once and then move on. You must – *I simply cannot stress this enough* – grow adept. However, you need not do them all. You should aim to succeed with ten out of the fifteen. The important thing is that you feel at ease: never attempt any if the idea upsets you. But be as adventurous as you dare. If you can do the lot you're a star pupil.

These fifteen methods are divided into four classes. The classes are simply a way of grouping together types of masturbation that make use of different skills. If you can think of others, which exploit new positions and new circumstances, then by all means try them too.

Of course, all women are different. Some of you may already be expert in some of the stages. The stages I have set out begin, roughly speaking, with the easier ways and progress to the more difficult and skilful. If you prefer, you may rearrange this part of the plan according to your ability.

I propose that you do each method at least five times before moving on to the next step of the programme. *But don't stop then.* You must keep learning, keep exploring, keep training.

If some of the methods I suggest are really beyond you (doing it in a public place, for example), or you can't succeed however hard you try, don't worry. Versatility can be acquired in many ways.

The important thing in each section is to *try* them. Time and again I have seen the look of horror on a woman's face when I have suggested some of the exercises, only to find that when she actually tried it she enjoyed it. Cassandra was typical:

> When I saw I was supposed to masturbate in semi-public I just collapsed. 'You can't be serious. It's a joke.' Rachel came straight back with: 'Fine, laugh as much as you like. It's good for you. *But do it.* It's not so outrageous.' So I did. And she's right. It's no big deal – and the exercises work, I promise you.

If you don't reach orgasm, don't worry. Continue, relishing whatever pleasure you do get.

CLASS A: MASTURBATION IN PRIVATE

Exercise 7.1 Lying down on the bed: on your back, using your hands. This is the basic skill, discussed at length above. Make sure, as with all the methods of class A, that there is no risk of you being disturbed, that you do not feel hurried, and you can devote your full attention to the task. Do this first with your clothes off. Then do it with your clothes on, by slipping your fingers into your underpants, and gaining direct contact. As a third alternative try bringing yourself to orgasm simply by rubbing yourself through your trousers or knickers.

Exercise 7.2 Lying down on the bed: on your front or on your back (whichever you prefer) using an object. *Not* an object for insertion, but one for rubbing against, such as a rolled up sock or pillow, or pulling a sheet back and forth between your legs, or simply moving against the mattress. You can rub something against *you* or you can rub *yourself* against something. As for all the methods of this class, do it both with your clothes on and with them off, direct and indirect contact.

Exercise 7.3 Sitting up in bed: arrange yourself comfortably, sitting at the head of the bed, with your back against the head-rest or wall. Once again, use all the usual variations.

Exercise 7.4 Sitting up on a chair: at first use a comfortable chair, perhaps with your legs splayed over the padded arms. Next try sitting in an ordinary, hard chair. Usual variations.

Exercise 7.5 Lying down on the bed: on your front, using your hands. You may find that pillows help you to get comfortable. If so, use them. This is important for building up your ability to have an orgasm in less than ideal conditions. Again, learn how to do it with clothes on and clothes off, with direct contact and indirect contact. (This is a difficult one.)

Exercise 7.6 In the bath: if you have a shower attachment, turn it on while sitting in a full bath, and direct the stream of warm water between your legs. You may not reach orgasm, but see how much pleasure you can give yourself from this method alone. After this, try masturbating yourself to orgasm with your hands, still in the bathtub.

Exercise 7.7 Standing up: my friend Sasha first masturbated standing up out of necessity. She was walking round a picture gallery and stopped in front of an extremely arousing painting –

some voluptuous seventeenth-century woman in an intimate situation with a man. She simply had to satisfy herself, so hurried down to the gallery's ladies room and locked herself in a cubicle. Wishing she was at home and not having to put up with such lousy circumstances, she lifted her skirt. Leaving her knickers on, she inserted her fingers still standing and began. It took a while for her to climax, but when she did

> **My God, I was nearly knocked backwards. Standing up,
> the pleasure travels all the way down both legs, like an
> electric charge seeking earth. A pretty good consolation for
> an otherwise not wildly comfortable position.**

So there you are: if you've never done it standing up before, try it leaning against a wall. Progress to all the usual variations.

Exercise 7.8 Squatting down, kneeling: quite a difficult one. Try this both against a wall, and in the middle of the room. Usual variations.

Exercise 7.9 Let your imagination run free: if you've got this far, you're really on the way. Now as well as variations of position, I suggest variations of speed. Try a slow session, long and drawn out lasting double or treble your usual time, all the while holding back your orgasm. This teaches you control. Now try to climax as quickly as possible. Try doing it twice in a row. See if you can do it twice within ten minutes. Try to do it as many times as possible, and keep a note of your record. Remember it is part of the sexual pleasures of being a woman that not only can we have numerous orgasms in one afternoon, but that we can do it without fuss or mess. Learn to develop and exploit these advantages.

Exercise 7.10 Masturbation with a dildo-like object inserted at the climax: for this you should masturbate in your usual manner, using only your hands, but have some sort of 'dildo' handy – it can be a vibrator, a banana, a candle, whatever you feel happiest with.

Then, just at the moment of orgasm you should insert the dildo, so that you enjoy the unique sensation of climaxing around something.

Exercise 7.11 Masturbation using a 'dildo' at all stages: this exercise speaks for itself. Basically I want you to try to masturbate yourself using your chosen dildo-type object as a penis – that is, moving it in and out. I personally cannot climax this way, without some help from my hands, even though I *can* do so with a man – perhaps because the angle of the man's body provides some of the necessary clitoral friction. You may have more success.

CLASS B: MASTURBATION IN SEMI-PUBLIC

Exercise 7.12 Masturbation in semi-public: the ideal place to begin this stage is the ladies room at work, or possibly the cloakroom of a museum or of a train. Nobody can break into your cubicle, but you might have the thrill of hearing people coming and going next door. You must remember, also, that however discreet you are with your hand movements, your breathing may give you away. After all, you don't want to be cosily tucked away in the office toilet and be disturbed by your boss knocking on the door to ask if you have been taken ill and need some brandy.

Now progress to doing it under your desk at work or in the library. Don't faint at the very idea. Nobody will know you are doing it – it will be a totally private action. All you need to do is exert a little pressure in the right place. You can use a book or your handbag: be inventive. You can always stop if it gets too dangerous. You'll find it a great deal of fun, and surprisingly easy on days when you're feeling especially horny. I used to do it in the cinema, where I could unzip my trousers unobserved. Best of all if it's a sexy film. Even if you can't actually bring yourself to orgasm at first – keep trying.

This is not simply a flippant exercise. It is an important part of the plan that you get accustomed to relaxing sufficiently to enjoy orgasm in situations that involve others. It is part of the process of breaking down that invisible barrier between you alone and you with somebody else.

CLASS C: MASTURBATION IN PUBLIC!

Exercise 7.13   For the really daring: if you can do this at will, then you're a star pupil. Of course nobody will know what you're doing. The trick is to exert some pressure where it matters, without seeming to be doing so. I've done it on the tube with my handbag timed to the rhythm of the train. More than once I've taken my cue from Laurelle, and used my heel while kneeling on the floor talking about the state of the nation. But if you're at this stage, you don't need me to point out the possibilities. If you really can't face it, don't. The truly important thing is to manage with ease the methods up to this point.

CLASS D: IMPROVING YOUR TIMING

These exercises simply concentrate on your timing.

Exercise 7.14   How many times in a row can you masturbate? Use your favourite position. At first it won't be more than once or twice. Later you'll progress – I know one woman whose record was thirteen times in one session. I thought that was pretty good going, but I recently read of another woman who managed 134! Beat that!

Exercise 7.15   How quickly can you masturbate? At first you'll be slow. Later you'll succeed in under ten minutes, and when you're really good you'll be able to come in a very short time indeed. This exercise depends a great deal on how horny you're feeling to begin with.

The Golden Rule is: KEEP IT UP. As you progress through the rest of the programme you *must* continue to practise, improve and vary your masturbation repertoire.

CHAPTER EIGHT

STEP 3: INTIMACY WITHOUT ORGASM

By thoroughly mastering step 2 you've made excellent progress. You will have greatly increased your control and understanding of your own sexuality. This constitutes a major advance towards your goal – don't let go of it! The lessons learned in step 2 should be regularly rehearsed so that they give the best support for your progress through the remaining steps. Keep practising masturbation in the old positions and circumstances, and build on your skills by continuing to invent new ones.

Step 3 provides the link between having an orgasm on your own and having one with the aid of a penis. How does it do this? Quite simply by insisting that you don't bother about orgasm at all. Just as in step 1, I want you to concentrate only on the feeling of non-orgasmic pleasure you can derive from sexual activity.

The advantage of this stage is that while it is sometimes difficult to initiate intimacy without orgasm, once it becomes a regular feature of your relationship he won't want to give it up.

SEXUAL RELAXATION

Don't we all remember the following scene? It's been a tiring day, you feel worn out and run down. Your boss has snapped at you, the supermarket has run out of a vital ingredient for supper tonight, and to crown it all the phone rings just as you step into the shower. Your partner is due any minute. You are looking forward to a quiet evening of affectionate intimacy and understanding.

For a while things go fine. You embrace. You sit down to a tempting meal. He compliments you on the food, you bring on the sorbet. The wine is helping you relax, but you're still a little edgy. You both move to the sofa, he puts his arms around you, nuzzles up to your neck and lightly strokes the neckline of your dress. Very pleasant.

But all too soon those little gestures of affectionate physical contact become *foreplay*. You wanted to have emotional comfort and the security of physical closeness, yet it quickly becomes a matter of sex. And sex of course concerns orgasm.

The evening may end in one of several ways: either you get mad and have a row; or you tense up, he doesn't notice, you go to bed, he has a whacking great orgasm and you feel foul; or you both tense up, you have sex, and neither of you enjoys it.

I have great sympathy. Maddening though my first husband could be, he was gentle in bed. After we split up it was a shock to find out that this quality is rather rare, and that too many men seemed to be the 'quick unzip, fumble and shove' type. I, who was wanting a warm, sympathetic relationship, felt that genuine intimacy was impossible. As far as my lovers were concerned there seemed only two types of closeness – nice, consoling chats about what to buy for supper, and a good screw. Nothing in between. This disheartening period of my life made me realize that however enjoyable you find sex there are times when the *inevitability* of it is distressing – times when one wants sexual understanding and appreciation without the passion and demands for penetration and climax.

So for this step I want you to establish intimate situations with your partner in which, before you even begin anything, there is no question of penetration and orgasm. These situations can be of two types: either occurring during special times set aside by mutual consent, or as a result of incidental encounters between the two of you whenever mood and occasion warrant them.

There are three great advantages to these situations: first, by eliminating even the possibility of orgasm they encourage mental relaxation for you, and help to put you at your ease about your ability to have an orgasm. Learning to relax during sexual encounters is a crucial part of learning how to have or improve your ability to have an orgasm. Second, such situations tend to be more gentle, slow and appreciative than intercourse, and this will help you to grow increasingly at ease with both your sexuality and his. Finally, they help develop a sense of control and sexual self-esteem, because *you* are employing the man for *your* purposes.

SETTING ASIDE A SPECIAL TIME

If you have an understanding partner it is worth asking him outright for such a session. Arrange a period of about thirty minutes to an hour when you can lie down together on the bed undisturbed. At first do this when you are both dressed. Explore each other's bodies, pass your hands under each other's clothes, but do not concentrate on the genital region. Caress, touch, massage, kiss, rub, stroke, play, snuggle up, murmur sweet nothings, hug, entwine, fondle – do it continuously or do it intermittently while you talk about other things. Be physically intimate however you like, but do not progress to penetration or to orgasm for either of you.

Try to establish this sort of involvement as something usual in your relationship. After a few such encounters start taking off each other's clothes. In order to ensure that you don't go too far, it's a good idea to begin such sessions just before an important engagement like a party, meeting or picking up the children from school. Obviously it's not something you want to do to the exclusion of full sex altogether, but it is a form of restrained contact that you should try to establish as common. Do it as often as you feel comfortable.

Even if, after a few minutes, you find that you would like to progress to intercourse, *don't*. You must be strict with both yourself and with him. If you feel that he may be able to bring you to orgasm this time without intercourse, or that you would like to try, or he seems to be getting it into his head that he'll make you climax, STOP. Thoughts about orgasm during these sessions are not only to be avoided, they are forbidden. These are purely times of relaxed intimacy.

The main difficulty with planned encounters is not so much *your* desire as *his*. Men are not used to such things; they tend to make the mistake of thinking that penetration (followed by their orgasm) is the goal of any sexual circumstance. Even if your partner does not, or you manage to enlighten him and free him from his prejudice, *you* may continue to worry that *he's* still wanting to get on with it. Or you may feel the very fact that the situation lays so much emphasis on lack of orgasm, that orgasm continues to be a disturbing issue.

There are a number of ways you can deal with this problem. Since the important thing about this step is that *you* do not feel you are expected to have an orgasm, you can make him climax before you begin the exercise. That over with, go on as before. Not only does he owe you the attention you demand, more importantly your worries about satisfying his desire have been removed. Alternatively you can make it clear that if he does this step with you as required, you'll satisfy his needs later in the day. The better he does it now, the greater his attention and expertise, the nicer his reward. Bargains are annoying in sex, but realistically speaking they can be useful. As Ovid remarked, 'Bribes, believe me, buy both gods and men.'

Lastly, even if you have successfully arranged and agreed upon sessions, don't skip the following – unplanned encounters can be extremely arousing.

UNPLANNED ENCOUNTERS

If you do not have a sympathetic partner then you may have to rely on your own ingenuity to create situations where you can have intimacy without orgasm. It probably won't be easy to set up special sessions. If it is, then have them whenever you can. But in either case, you should also take advantage of situations which have not been specially planned; with a little subterfuge you can arrange them fairly frequently.

Fiona tells her story:

> I didn't feel I could ask Alan for arranged sessions. At first I was quite stumped as to what to do – then I thought of the television. I waited till I knew there was a film he was really eager to see, then set to work. All the while he was engrossed in *Death on the Nile* I had my hands round his prick, and I made sure he had his in my knickers. It's all a question of getting the balance right: he must like doing the two things equally. A detective film's the best, because he daren't get too carried away or he misses the plot.

The best way, as before, is to begin arousing him just before you have to do something important. If you're both about to go to a party in the evening, wait till he's bathed and shaved before you start to feel around. It needn't last long, but it must be understood that if things progress too far you'll miss the event. For this reason a dinner party engagement is obviously better than an ordinary drinks party, as there's not so much scope for being late. If possible, continue to give and receive a little more sexual attention during the party: under the table in the semi-darkness. But again, there should be no prospect of orgasm. Or take advantage of the darkness in a cinema or theatre, or on a train at night.

Perhaps the best thing I've discovered is getting my partner to attend to me while I'm driving. He rubs between my legs and along my thighs as he sits in the passenger seat – his life depends on my *not* having an orgasm.

Ideally, you are ready to progress to the next stage when you have managed to introduce these non-orgasmic situations as a familiar and accepted part of your normal sex life. But you may move on sooner, once you have learnt to accept them yourself as something reasonable and enjoyable without guilt or tension.

As an added bonus I might point out that I've found such unplanned encounters *unfailingly* popular with men, and the end result is usually greater willingness to do what *you* want. For this reason I think you'll find that these escapades – especially those that take place outside of the home – will become a permanent feature of your relationship.

CHAPTER NINE

STEP 4: MASTURBATION WITH A PENIS

Now that you are thoroughly familiar with masturbation, it is time to progress to step 4. For this stage you *will* need a partner. Either (as we discussed before) a willing and compliant partner, or a partner who remains in blissful ignorance of the fact that you are in the midst of a training programme.

The idea is to develop your new-found versatility, to use it as a stepping stone to obtaining orgasm *in coitus*. Put simply, in this chapter you will learn – in four stages of increasing penile involvement – to masturbate with a penis.

Step 4 is the pivotal stage in breaking through that invisible barrier, because in it you are getting accustomed to the idea of another person, while still retaining essential control.

As with all stages in this programme, it is important that you are thoroughly comfortable and relaxed. Therefore, as before, spend a little thought in setting the scene first. Read through Chapter 5 on 'Preparing for Orgasm'. Decide what you will wear during the evening, and later in bed. Adjust the lighting in your bedroom so that you are quite comfortable with it. If you feel comfortable you will feel relaxed.

THE STARFISH POSITION

Some years ago I was invited to a book-launch party at a friend's house. I can't remember what the book was – a first novel probably, because there was a young man hanging about looking humourless and artifically bitter – but there was a lot to drink and the fun went on until quite late. Somehow I ended up with a very suave individual – and that night, thanks to a great deal of inventiveness on my part, the Starfish Position was born.

This is a sexual position that I have found to be ideal for the exercises in this step. I would like you to practise it – as far as you can – alone at first. When you are thoroughly familiar with the idea of it, you can join with your partner.

Begin by making the bed comfortable.

Now lie on your back, with your partner to your right. He lies on his left-hand *side*. Then you lift your right leg up and slot his right leg beneath it and over the top of your left, so that his thigh crosses between your legs with his penis able to slip into you just beneath. It sounds hideously complicated in print, so I've included a diagram of it – in practice it's as easy as pie.

The Starfish Position has many advantages for the woman on this programme:

Step 4: Masturbation with a Penis

1. You are lying on your back in your *familiar masturbatory position*, so that you feel quite at home.

2. It is an extremely relaxing position, physically, because you are not having to support yourself or your partner. It is also versatile: try it out and you will see that while retaining the essential position, all kinds of slight variations are possible.

3. It is mentally relaxing, and allows you plenty of freedom to concentrate on your own needs. The only essential point of contact with your partner is the genital region. Because he is lying off to one side he need not gaze into your face, which frees you from the obligation to 'look' a certain way – beautiful, enticing, loving or obviously aroused. *Don't underestimate the distracting power of this kind of thing.* Furthermore, you do not have the 'diversion' of kissing, and the other usual attentions of sex – of course these are all an integral part of making love, but at this stage of your learning they can disrupt the task in hand. On the other hand if you do wish to kiss and fondle, it is quite possible to do so by simply manoeuvring your torsos closer together.

4. It is the *most private* position, allowing you great independence, and freedom from embarrassment. If you're shy about your body, you can pull the bedclothes up around you.

5. It allows you *free access* to your own genitalia – you may rub yourself without impediment and probably without your partner knowing that you are doing so. This depends on precisely how you arrange his leg across yours.

6. His leg serves as a means of providing pressure *where you want it*. It is easy to adjust the position slightly, here and there, without too much disruption.

7. It is difficult for the man to insist on his pace. If he does try to outrun you, exert pressure from your legs to slow him down. If you want to speed him up, try moving your hips.

8. Last but not least, the Starfish is an excellent way of getting sex from a sleepy or drunk partner who looks like collapsing. His active involvement is minimal, and the position is remarkably comfortable.

In short, the Starfish Position gives you the means to be entirely in control of the situation, and of yourself. I found it was ideal for the progression from masturbation to intercourse. In fact, after I had recommended it to a number of women I found that there were even more unexpected advantages. Susan explains:

> I use it most in the mornings. You wake up, feeling sleepy and lazy, you haven't brushed your teeth, the remains of last night's mascara may well be creeping where it shouldn't, but you're as horny as a unicorn . . . Neither of you has the energy to climb on top. You just sidle up to each other and Bob's your uncle! After all, you don't always feel like the full kissing nonsense first thing in the morning!

I personally think it's perfect for the morning after the night before, when you've probably got a bit of a hangover. If you decide that the guy you met last night doesn't look so good in daylight, you can still get him to please you without all the intimacy.

Alexandra was having trouble with her husband. Not because she couldn't climax, but because she just felt *bored* with sex. I suggested she try this position for a bit of variety. Three weeks later she wrote to me:

> The Starfish is great, and I don't just mean for the reasons you gave me. I got my husband to try it, simply as a new position to give a bit of pep to our lovemaking. What you didn't tell me is that the type of pressure exerted on my pussy is unique. A sort of gentle *nudging*. Not insistent at all, and so mild that I hardly noticed it at first . . . Never mind his penis going in and out like a piston, it's the soft bumping against my fanny that makes me come. We do it all the time now.

All in all I have not, to date, come across another position which provides so many of the private advantages of masturbation, but also allows for maximum stimulation of both partners *in coitus*.

However, it is not essential that you use the Starfish for the exercises in step 3. I *recommend* that you do so, but I don't insist.

What I do insist on is that you give it a try. Don't dismiss it out of hand. It's far too valuable for that.

STAGE ONE: EXCITING YOURSELF WITH HIS PENIS

The first stage is to pursue your normal masturbation, but with a small amount of penile involvement. You are going to practise stimulating your clitoris, and the area around it, with the head of his penis. Just think of it as another example of masturbating with an object, as discussed in the last chapter, only in the place of a sock or a teddy bear you're now using a penis.

The following instructions are given on the assumption that you are both in the Starfish Position. If for any reason you are not, you must be inventive in adapting yourself to the circumstances.

Instead of inserting his penis right into you, have him rest it just inside the lips of your vagina. Then reach down between your own legs and gently grasp the shaft of the penis. Rub the head of it softly back and forth around your clitoris and the entrance to your vagina. You will find this a very delicious feeling, for the head of the penis is the softest, gentlest part. *Do not* attempt penetration. And don't even think about orgasm; just lie back and enjoy the pleasurable sensations this manipulation produces.

After you have been doing this for a while, bring your own hands into play, and try to bring yourself to orgasm in the usual masturbatory way that is familiar to you. But even if your own hands are doing most of the work, don't lose hold of his penis. If you find that you cannot keep hold of it, or it is too distracting for you to do both – don't worry. It doesn't matter in the least. Simply continue and practise this step until you are able to bring yourself to orgasm *with the help of the penis*. However long it takes, continue until you have achieved this.

While you are exciting yourself with his penis, try to think of it as no more than an extension of your solitary masturbation sessions. As far as possible forget about him. If this sounds sacrilegious, all I can say is that this is a means to enable you to love and appreciate him tenfold. For the moment you must think of yourself.

And what's he doing all this while? Encourage him to lie back, close his eyes and relax altogether. Perhaps ply him with a drink beforehand. If he gets restless, moisten your hand and at the same time as you are pleasuring yourself, contrive to rub the shaft of the penis itself. This should ensure his enjoyment, especially as he is having to do none of the work. If this technique is new to your partner, you may well simply have to be inventive in how you initiate it. Jessica's husband was a very traditional sort, with reservations about anything new. She cured him of that by taking him to a blue movie, and later, when he was feeling weak, suggested they try some of the positions they'd just been watching. Which, of course, led on to trying the positions *she* wanted. In fact it's usually enough just to make it quite clear that you enjoy it. If not, I find that, contrary to the popular saying, flattery gets you *everywhere*. Try something like, 'Your penis is so attractive, but I never get to really *feel* the head.'

This stage has a special benefit for you because as the shaft of the penis is not employed there is much less risk of the man ejaculating before you are ready. The very knowledge of this should reassure you, as we all know how off-putting it is when we feel that your partner is about to come too soon.

A very sleepy man is useful in this respect. If he comes home and collapses on the bed, take advantage. Get undressed, sidle into bed with him, and ever so quietly remove his trousers. Now massage his penis until it is sufficiently erect to be of some use to you. With a little ingenuity you should be able to manoeuvre yourself into position. Now lie back and have fun.

Jacqueline quickly became an expert.

> The first time I tried this method it was as good as masturbating, only I got an extra kick because as well as using a real penis *I* was the one fully in control . . . The trouble was, I got to like it so much that I had to think of ways of getting Pete immobile. Before then I used to get really angry when he got drunk and fell on the bed.

Nowadays I'm always plying him with drinks, and when we go to parties together I usually offer to drive home, so he need have no inhibitions . . . Once we get home I slide into bed beside him, open my legs, and rub myself with his prick.

Louise finds that this method works well on those occasions when she's suffering from insomnia and he's not. 'Very few men will object to being woken in the night for this sort of treatment,' she insists, as long as you don't choose a night when he's got to get up early the next morning.

If you find you cannot climax, it is probably because the penis – being attached to a hunk of man – has not quite the same flexibility as your usual masturbatory tool. (Hubby is not so obliging as Teddy.) Never mind. Transfer the penis to your other hand and masturbate yourself in the usual way. Do it just as you have been practising. It's now that your rigid programme of masturbation practice comes in really useful. You must start learning to achieve orgasm with the *help* of his penis. It doesn't matter if his penis does not do much of the work – just masturbate with your own hand as you are used to doing. But make sure the penis is somewhere nearby.

The important thing is that gradually you are developing from pure masturbation into a sex-with-partner situation. And because you are learning, practising and cementing each stage as you go, you are teaching yourself a skill that you will not lose.

Continue until you are adept at this stage.

STAGE TWO: HAVING AN ORGASM WITH A PENIS

The next stage is to introduce a little more penile involvement. You will bring yourself to orgasm, either as above or in your normal masturbatory way, and as you climax *insert your partner's penis into your vagina*. This is a parallel to Exercise 7.10 in the chapter on masturbation. Get yourself and your partner all set up, as before. As you rub yourself make sure the penis is nearby. The moment you feel yourself go beyond the limit – that wonderful uphill surge towards orgasm – manoeuvre yourself on to his penis as far as you can. Even just a little will do; it needn't go in all the way. As you come, savour the sensations of your vagina contracting around it.

Congratulations! This is one more vital step in breaking down that invisible barrier between orgasm alone and orgasm with a man. If you can establish a situation of penis-related orgasm, followed by his penetration, then you are well on the way to full acceptance of him. But it's not enough to do it once. You must practise until it is no longer a hit-and-miss affair, but something you *know* you can do.

Remember, as always, it is essential that you do not neglect your private masturbatory programme. If you have a set-back with this stage, never mind. Return to step 2 and *practise, practise, practise*. It'll come right in the end.

If step 4 is occupying all your nights (although there's no need for this – as I said earlier, you should ensure the plan fits into your usual sex life in the most convenient, least stressful way, not that it takes over), continue practising step 2 during the day. You must continue to improve and explore. With each new stage, you must make sure that your learning is backed up by appropriate skills in private masturbation.

Now that you are so far along, and you are beginning to become an advanced pupil, you should continue to masturbate with an object for insertion.

STAGE THREE: MASTURBATING WITH AN IMMOBILE PENIS

Now is the time to make a significant advance. You are going to encourage the man to insert his penis gently *all the way in*. Let him lie quite still, while you gradually masturbate to orgasm in whatever way you find most effective. This will probably be rubbing yourself just above the clitoris, as other types of access will be restricted by his penis.

Of all the stages of step 4 this is the most important, and it is worth spending some time to perfect it. In fact some women (those with highly unco-operative partners) have found that it is the only stage out of step 4 that they need to do. I personally find it the most enjoyable, and once you've initiated it with a man he usually falls for it too. As Gina pointed out:

> It's a dead easy way for him to prolong sex before he ejaculates, so he doesn't have to feel guilty about being a trigger-happy male. He can do it in any way he likes without having to worry about giving me enough clitoral stimulation after I've had my go. It's ace. Much more intimate.

The Starfish Position is, of course, ideal because it leaves you freedom to move your hands. On the other hand, if your partner is on top of you, in the Missionary Position, it is still relatively easy to reach down. Obviously you will have to encourage him to stay still.

Simply continue to masturbate yourself in whatever way you like, until you climax – however long it takes you. It is an *extremely* pleasurable feeling.

> Thomas likes to give 'a helping hand'. He says he finds it really sexy to reach down, sometimes holding my hand as I'm doing it and following the movements. I think it can be quite helpful, too, not only because it means that you're both playing an active role but because it makes your partner's involvement greater – breaking down the barrier and all that. I'm slower when he helps, because I still feel a bit embarrassed, but I'm much easier about it than I used to be.

STAGE FOUR: MASTURBATING WITH A MOVING PENIS

Now that you have succeeded in climaxing with his penis immobile inside you, encourage him to have intercourse with you gently *while you masturbate*. It is a sort of double act: he moves slowly in and out while you rub yourself.

Once again you may find it helpful to forget that you are with a partner. Relax, close your eyes, and think that you are alone, practising one of the masturbation exercises of step 2. The importance of step 4 is that it appears sufficiently close to step 2 (masturbation) to seem but a small progression, and therefore a very possible one.

You may wish to stop him now and again – either to prevent him reaching orgasm too soon, or to catch up yourself. If you have difficulty, try a different position. At this stage the important thing about positions is that they give easy access and are comfortable. Later on, when you are more accomplished, you will think of positions as exciting ways to expand your sex life.

Thelma, who helped me to do some research for Chapter 16, offered the following advice:

> At first the problem was that Ray always came too soon. But I quickly realized that I *enjoyed* this. We begin by my rubbing myself while he moves in and out. After he's come he just stays there in me. I go on rubbing myself until I come – which I always do quite quickly. It's a halfway house between this stage and the previous stage, but a good one. Often, I think, you'll find that the mere fact that you don't have to worry at all about his timing any more can greatly help you with your own.

If, despite trying a variety of positions, you still have difficulty, don't worry. It takes time. It will get better. Hite reports that of women who do orgasm readily, most require direct clitoral stimulation. Persevere with the plan and you will get past this stage as well. Clitoral stimulation is something both of you can easily work on to improve, as the next steps explain. But for the moment recognize that you have come a long way.

You are well on the road to success.

A WORD OF ADVICE

I am well aware that the four separate stages of step 4 may seem confusing at first. Trying to put physical actions into words always appears to add complications. In fact they are very simple. When you are familiar with the programme, and have read it through once or twice, these will clarify themselves.

As I have already said, in a sense step 4 is the crucial part of the whole programme, because it brings together two situations: sex without a penis and sex with a penis. For this reason it will probably take longer than the other steps. Practise each stage fully until you are thoroughly familiar with them and they are no longer hit-and-miss affairs.

Ideally you should aim to accomplish the four stages as I have set them out. But only if you can do so easily. If your partner is unco-operative, it's far more important that you take advantage of natural situations as they present themselves. Just don't give in too easily!

Therefore, if you have the opportunity for stage 4 don't throw it up just because you haven't accomplished stage 3. Be flexible. To perfect each stage, so that you are *certain* that you can achieve it is more important than the order of the stages. And, if your options for this step are really limited, confine yourself to stage 3.

And remember, just as with the other steps, once you have completed this one, *don't* forget about it. Keep making sure that you continue now and then to bring yourself to climax in the ways suggested here.

HOW DO I GET MY PARTNER TO CO-OPERATE IN STEP 4?

This, of course, is the million-dollar question. So let's divide the answer into six possible categories:

1. Request
2. Suggestion
3. Guile
4. Bribery or bargaining
5. Threats
6. Give up and find yourself a new man

1. Requesting is straightforward. If you have a good relationship, sexual openness can only benefit you both. The only debatable point is do you reveal *why* you want to do it this way, or do you simply say you like it, full stop. That's up to you. My advice is if you feel uncertain keep your plans to yourself for now. You can always reveal your intentions later. I think it's better to feel quite comfortable about your progress in the programme before you bring him in, if you have any suspicions that his involvement might not always be helpful.

2. By suggestion I mean lots of 'Mmmmms' and 'Aaaaahhs' when you 'happen' to find yourself in the position you want. So he puts two and two together and thinks he's discovered a way to seem a great lover: before you know it he's suggesting it himself.

3. By guile I mean such wiles as manipulating a drunk or sleepy partner.

4. Bribery or bargaining involves a swap – you agree to do such and such if he agrees to the position you want. As I've already mentioned, not ideal but definitely not to be sneezed at for tricky situations. Handled with a bit of subtlety, it can be made into a personal joke between you.

5. By threats, I mean threats to walk out on him/go home to mother/run off with the next-door neighbour, etc. This may sound alarming, but if he so doggedly refuses to help with what gives you special pleasure, then you're justified. Besides, you may find that if you really stand your ground he'll give in, especially if you've never tested him that far before.

6. Option 6 is the most drastic of all, but it might actually be your best bet. If agreeing about something so fundamental to a relationship as sex is impossible, ask yourself what you *do* have going for you as a couple. Quite frankly, if he's not prepared to be a little accommodating to your needs then you don't have a great future together. Sounds brutal? Ask yourself: Would he keep *me* on if I didn't give *him* what he wants? If the answer is 'no', *don't hesitate to set the same standards for yourself.*

CHAPTER TEN

STEP 5: INTERCOURSE

Now you are going to attempt to have an orgasm with you partner's penis inside you, but without masturbating yourself.

In theory this is a big step. In practice it's a small and manageable progression. Firstly, by continual exercise and learning you have been gradually narrowing the gap between this and the last step. Secondly, by virtue of having had to train your body and its sexuality up to this point, you have become much more understanding of your needs, and in control of your responses.

Remember, at this stage you are still not expecting orgasm to happen immediately. Just as you practised and practised steps 2, 3 and 4, so you must thoroughly practise step 5 until you succeed. And, as always, you must support your programme by continually repeating and improving on your earlier successes of the last two steps.

Once again you must prepare carefully. Take out your pen and paper and think hard: what inhibiting factors are there in your lovemaking? Be ruthless: write them *all* down and think about how to correct them. Are you still making little concessions to *his* pleasure at the expense of your own ease?

It's not easy to identify inhibiting factors. Sometimes they're so subconscious we can't spot them at all, yet they spoil our pleasure. With practice your self-awareness will increase. And when you do come across something that bothers you, put a stop to it. Or try striking a balance, even if you have to invent something he does that annoys you. *Selfishness* is all-important – at least for the time being – and that is a thing many women find difficult to exercise in the bedroom.

Lorna, for example, was making good progress in the programme, but she was conscious of a nagging anxiety. After careful thought she realized that she always felt slightly self-conscious with the light on.

> It wasn't a significant thing, really. I mean I wasn't messed up about it. My figure's not bad, but I have stretchmarks all round my stomach and thighs. Mark's told me loads of times that he doesn't mind, and the crazy thing is I even believe him. But they went on bothering me. I *knew* I wasn't 100 per cent relaxed. Problem was, Mark said he hated making love in the dark. Sometimes I simply insisted we turn the light off, but it made me feel mean and therefore I couldn't relax then either. So I evolved a plan where I simply made love clothed – either partially or fully. I bought one of those sexy all-in-one garments made of black Lycra stretchy stuff. It undid at the crotch. Now if Mark wants the light on I wear that. He unbuttons the buttons and of course I *have* to keep it on, that's part of the pleasure. So we're both satisfied. He seemed to find that a real turn on. It gave me a lot of confidence.

Light is a very common anxiety – and not only because we worry about our bodies. I once made the mistake of faking a really strong orgasm with a boyfriend when he was feeling low about his work, just to give him a boost. He came home one sunny afternoon and was moping about the flat. I felt sorry for him and I inveigled him into bed. His lovemaking was no great shakes at the best of times, but I would've earned an Oscar for my performance. My artifice did wonders for his morale (he was promoted a month later) but nearly destroyed mine, because it gave him a disconcerting desire to watch my face so he could see how much satisfaction he'd given me. After that he started insisting that we made love with the light on. In those days I hadn't learned to be inventive. It killed my desire stone dead.

Suzy was worried about the noises she made during sex.

> I couldn't help it; if I was enjoying the sex I'd make a noise – groans and moans. I was so embarrassed about it. For one thing we lived in a pre-fab bungalow and the walls were really thin. Our next-door neighbour used to give me some looks. I also worried that Pete would think me disgusting and farm-yardish, but I couldn't stop. I put the radio on, but that never worked because quite often half my mind would be on what the DJ was saying. Once in desperation I even tried chewing gum, but Pete objected (can't say I blame him). Then one day he put his hand in my mouth, and instead of making noises, I sort of sucked and bit on that. I began to feel his fingers probing around my tongue and lips, and pushing in and out – he was too excited to notice until after. We do that quite often now. Otherwise I use my own hand, or the edge of a pillow, and I try and make sure I have him in positions which make this gesture less obvious.

While on the subject of noise, let me say that the *Kama Sutra* takes it very seriously and lists eight classes of sound that women utter during sexual pleasure: hin, thundering, cooing, weeping, phut, phat, sut and plat. So next time, instead of feeling self-conscious, try to work out which category yours falls into . . .

WHICH POSITION?

Once you are quite certain about details such as lighting, clothing, etc., it is time to consider which sexual position you are going to employ for step 5. Here are just a few comments on the suitability of the sexual positions for the plan. I have deliberately included only the standard ones (with, of course, the exception of the

Starfish) for the simple reason that these work best for orgasm. It is another outrageous sex myth that bizarre and exotic positions equal explosive sex. They may do for someone highly experienced in orgasm, and they probably give pep to a routine-bound sex life. But for a woman wanting to improve her orgasm skills they can be fatal. Besides, you'd have to be double-jointed to manage some of them. A curiously large number of the ancient oriental guides to sophisticated lovemaking were written or painted with a complete disregard for human anatomy. Unless you can devise a position that for some reason particularly suits you, my advice is stick to the basics.

The Missionary Position

The Missionary Position has long been out of fashion. 'Boring', 'old-fashioned', 'redolent of male dominance' are just some of the descriptions used to denigrate this old favourite. Personally, I'm a great believer in it, at least for the early learning stages of step 5. It is extremely comfortable for the woman, who (unless the man is very large indeed) can lie back without the need to support herself. And it is comfortably close to the familiar masturbatory position you have been practising. You need have few worries about your figure, as you will be largely covered by your partner.

Also, it is not simply the *insertion* of the penis that is pleasurable, but the clitoral stimulation. It is in this position that the angle between the man's body and his penis is such that his pelvis can rub against your genital region where it is most effective. Only in rare cases – such as Joyce's – is this undesirable:

> It's all in, out, in, out, and not enough shake-it-all-about with Simon. All the concentration, in other words, is on my vagina, and the result is that not enough gets to my clitoris. I wish he'd slow down a little and not plunge quite so much, but spend more time moving his hips over me and putting pressure where my clitoris is.

Another slight disadvantage is that your partner controls the rhythm and pace.

If you are in the Missionary Position and finding it difficult to climax, try this: using either both hands or just one, clasp your partner round the buttocks as if it were you who is causing him to move in and out. Firstly you will be modifying his rhythm and pace to suit yourself. But, more importantly, it gives an excellent *illusion* that you are in control. The fact of your seeming to use him as a tool puts you back in the familiar and reassuring position of masturbation – that is, you controlling yourself, rather than someone else controlling you. Again and again this tip has helped women who are having trouble climaxing.

TWO IMPORTANT VARIANTS OF THE MISSIONARY POSITION

Man raised If your partner, instead of simply lying on top of you, pushes his body up above you slightly by resting on his elbows or (if he's got the strength and inclination) on his outstretched arms, this will put greater pressure on the clitoral region. This may require a bit of experiment to get it right, because too much pressure can be painful on the skin, both for you and for him. But once you succeed you'll soon realize the benefits.

Man on top with legs apart Instead of his legs between yours, try it the other way round, with you keeping your legs together and he opening his. As with 'man raised' this is a useful variant because it provides a good deal of friction on the area around the clitoris.

Woman on top

Many sex therapists suggest that for women who find it difficult to climax this position is helpful. I don't necessarily agree – it depends very much on your circumstances. Being on top gives the woman a certain amount of control: she does the rubbing, sets the pace and stops when she feels like it. And because *rhythm* is a crucial feature in learning to climax, this is important.

If by being on top you can really give yourself a sense of control, marvellous. But as the woman on top is something of a male fantasy, too often this position ends with the woman being manipulated by a lazy man to his own preferences. Don't let this happen. If necessary make an exaggerated play of dominance and control by pinning your lover's arms above his head, so that he *has* to submit. For Judy this is what gives her sex a certain frisson:

> I don't think I'd get any pleasure out of sex if I thought I was 'submitting'. I want him to know who's boss. I like to get on top, sink myself on to him, grind away for a few delectable minutes, then stop and deliberately watch him beg for more. Then I put my fists on his chest and lift up and down slowly, pumping him, so that his chest goes white with the pressure I'm putting on, but he doesn't dare move in case I stop moving. Sometimes I slap him. He tries to slap me back but I grab his arms and force them down. Also I can make him suck my tits, which sends shivers down my spine, like aah!

On the other hand there are certain disadvantages to the woman on top position. Thrusting up and down on top of a man can be very tiring indeed – moving more against gravity than a man on top would be. This is particularly true if, instead of lying on the man, the woman remains upright – as that infamous turn-of-the-century writer and Lothario Frank Harris here explains:

> She got up smiling and straddled kneeling across me, and put my cock in her pussy and sank down on me with a deep sigh. She tried to move up and down on my organ and at once came up too high and had to use her hand to put my Tommy in again; then she sank down on it as far as possible. 'I can sink down all right,' she cried, smiling at the double meaning, 'but I cannot rise so well!'

123

Sitting on the man has the added disadvantage of diminishing clitoral contact. This can be counteracted, of course, if he uses his hands, but otherwise it's only by lying on top and making sure of sufficient clitoral friction that you can get the necessary amount.

The woman on top may have the added distraction of having to support herself on her arms. And many women feel they must go to great lengths not to seem too heavy and 'unladylike'. The position can be actively uncomfortable in certain situations: for example, if the man is very skinny and the woman has long legs. In this case placing pillows beneath his bottom usually remedies the situation.

Above all, if you are self-conscious about your breasts, don't attempt it. However much *he* appreciates your assets, if *you* feel awkward about them then don't choose a position which puts them in the limelight. 'I used to feel I was a lone contender in a topless bathing contest,' remarked one woman. 'It made me nervous as hell.' It's little anxieties like this that can spoil your chance of orgasm. Later, when you are more accomplished, these details will no longer be so important.

The Starfish Position

The many advantages of this position have been discussed in Chapter 9, so I shall not repeat them here. I can only add that both of you have pretty equal control; neither one of you is 'dominant'. If you sense your partner is close to climaxing, you can pull out or stop. Also, it is the most private of the positions, and best if you feel sensitive or nervous about yourself.

Side by side

The Roman poet Ovid, who wrote copiously on the art of love, found this a great favourite:

There are a thousand modes of love; a simple one and least fatiguing is when the woman lies upon her right side, half inclined.

Though not an easy position to achieve, this has the advantage that it avoids the heavy and macho thrusting sometimes associated with the Missionary. It has another major advantage: because there is constant likelihood that the penis will slip out, you can ensure a very slow, careful pace. If your partner is a fiery stallion who won't slow down, try this one. There is, however, a reverse side to the coin: unlike women, men sometimes come much quicker if they're having sex in an unusual position, so you'll have to break him in. Furthermore, if he has to concentrate about keeping his penis in, this isn't much help for rhythm and your concentration.

Man enters from behind

In my experience women vary greatly in their opinions about this position. The most common response is 'I like it, but it's hard to climax this way' – because there is very little contact with the clitoris. In fact I know several women who have learned to climax readily in a variety of positions, but never in this one. Others, like Loretta, find it highly enjoyable:

I like the slight anonymity of this position. You can really feel the man, but you also feel unencumbered. I love Rob dearly, but sometimes I need the freedom of nobody in front of my face, watching me, bearing down on me. I do it with me kneeling and him kneeling behind me.

Netta has another slant:

What I like about it is it's a great means to make love in odd situations, without all the bother of getting undressed and into bed. I'll give you an example.

Jack and I were recently staying with friends in the country. It was a hot summer's day, they'd made a barbecue and we were all milling about feeling relaxed. Their garden is huge – lots of ponds, trees and bushes. I got fed up with chatting so I went for a walk. I'd just knelt down to look at some flowers when Jack came up behind me. He'd seen me slip away and followed. He lifted my skirt and began stroking between my legs. He didn't even bother to take my knickers off (I was worried someone might surprise us) but just pulled them aside and did it to me, while I carried on picking flowers. Definitely one of the best fucks I've ever had. I could see the rest of the party through the hedge.

This position has all the obvious advantages of privacy, but it's not so good on control. You can, however, reach behind and hold his hips if you need to. It has the obvious disadvantage of making your bottom the focal point, although it's worth pointing out that in a kneeling position all bottoms – unlike breasts – look pretty much alike, so this shouldn't put you off!

You might find with appropriate masturbatory practice that this position becomes more satisfying, particularly if you put a pillow beneath you to enhance the friction. Some women, I know, can have an orgasm this way, although I've never managed it myself.

MY PARTNER'S PENIS IS TOO SMALL!

I wonder just how many thousand times each year despairing women utter this exclamation. Perhaps understandably, many women who are unable to climax feel that their lack of success must be due to the size of their partner's organ. I have to admit I'm tempted to answer, 'Yes, only with a great whopper can a woman be truly satisfied,' simply to reduce some egos a little – certain men seem absolutely obsessed with huge penises. That might make them a little less critical of women's sexual parts.

However, the general consensus seems to be that size makes little difference to a woman's ability to climax. So next time you're confronted with a modest little chippolata of a penis, don't despair. The vagina is very elastic and therefore accommodates itself nicely to organs large and small.

This *doesn't* mean, however, that individual women don't have distinct preferences. I for one make no apologies for saying that I prefer a good-sized article – circumcised if possible. It may not make you have a better orgasm, but it gives you a nice full feeling. On the other hand, one can feel affectionately protective towards a small penis. Men have the advantage that if they go for big-breasted women they can see what they're after before they commit themselves. Not so women if they happen to prefer a large penis – unless you're a nudist. And even then, a limp penis gives little indication of the size it'll eventually grow to.

But one thing that reading a lot of erotic literature will tell you – it's *men*, not women, who are obsessed with enormous plonkers. If you're not getting satisfied, it's far more likely to be how your partner is using his penis than how big it is. Besides, a too big one is downright uncomfortable.

The subject of different sized organs leads me on to another point. That is, that several women I've met succeeded in having an orgasm with a lover, where they had consistently failed with their husband (or regular partner). Since the organs in question were all pretty much the same size (and in two cases, the lovers' were smaller) this is good evidence that it's the use a penis is put to rather than its dimensions that counts.

In one case the relationship with the lover ended, and the woman felt uncomfortably guilty afterwards. I tried to encourage her to regard this lapse not as the end of the world, but as the beginning of a new life with her husband – a life with successful sex. Since the experience with the lover proved that she could climax, why not think of it as something positive for the husband too? I urged her *not* to confess: oh, how rarely are those confessions justified, most of the time they serve to make the guilty feel less guilty, while the innocent partner suffers. Instead, she put her attention into repeating the orgasm with her husband: a far smaller step than she originally thought. Remember, orgasms don't belong to the partner, they belong to *you*. And, if you have lapsed, what you learn with another man, you can offer to your permanent partner. The chances are, your sex life will improve so much that you won't want to do it again with someone else.

TWO VITAL INGREDIENTS OF SUCCESSFUL SEX

The two vital ingredients of successful sex for women who have trouble climaxing are often overlooked or taken for granted: namely *rhythm* and *concentration*. I have said again and again that in the early stages of learning to have an orgasm it is simply not enough to 'lie back and relax'. Until you are really proficient in achieving orgasm, you must put a little thought and effort into it.

Rhythm: the Snakes and Ladders principle

The man's failure to maintain a consistent and acceptable rhythm is one of the chief causes of women's failure to climax. Of all those I have spoken to about difficulty with orgasm, all agree that a consistent rhythm in the lead up to orgasm is crucial. If the rhythm is broken, then the gradual ascent to orgasm is also broken. Many of you will have discovered the use of rhythm while masturbating: there are days when one feels so horny that any pressure sends you off, but often as not to reach a climax you need to establish a steady *rhythm*.

Men are much the same, although in general less sensitive to changes: when you rub his penis with your hand you establish a rhythm he likes. The trouble is, in *coitus*, when he's doing the thrusting, it's *his* rhythm and not necessarily yours. Susan takes up the point:

> I've been in situations where I'm wild with desire. He tries all sorts of crazy things – does it hard, then soft, then very

slow – you name it. I've been so worked up I could scream. But if I want to actually *come* I have to get him to establish a consistent rhythm, a pace if you like, for at least five or ten minutes beforehand.

In fact Susan was so interested she called it the Snakes and Ladders principle.

I think of it like this: orgasm is to be found at the top of a long ladder. Each rung of the ladder is equally spaced and each rung represents a thrust of his penis – a steady rhythm. I can only get to the top of the ladder (orgasm) by going up each rung one at a time. You *must* have that even rhythm for the lead up. If he breaks the rhythm he jumps *you* on to a snake – and you go all the way down again. The funny thing is, if he does break the rhythm, I can still find it terribly sexy but I know I won't climax from it. Then you're torn between urging him on and begging him to go back to the original.

Of course I am not saying that this particular need for a consistent 'ladder rhythm' will apply to all women. Some of you may reach orgasm more readily from varied movements. But I have found that in the great majority of women still learning to be proficient in orgasm, this is the case. The more accomplished you become, the less the 'ladder rhythm' will matter.

Exercise 10.1 In order to fully understand rhythm, I want you to try the following. Begin masturbating *at a period when you don't feel particularly sexy*. As I mentioned above, when you feel very horny orgasm is readily obtained and the exercise will not help you with your difficulties. But if you have to work hard for your orgasm during masturbation, the chances are you'll have to find a rhythm. Work yourself up until you are close to climaxing: then stop and alter the rhythm. Do the same thing again, but this time lose the rhythm altogether, and simply rub yourself in a random fashion.

You'll soon begin to see the importance of rhythm – and more importantly to gauge the one that suits *you*. Then, when you go back to sex with your partner, be similarly conscious of which will help you best.

And just to show how important tempo can be, let me quote from Dr Sofie Lazarsfeld's *Woman's Experience of the Male*:

> We are reminded of the popular custom in Thuringia. There a couple will not marry until the boy and girl have sawn through a log together. If the rhythm of their movements agrees, the marriage takes place, otherwise the association is broken off.

The essential partner to rhythm in achieving orgasm is *concentration*.

Concentration

Believe it or not concentration and relaxation are companions, not opposites. We are all aware of how many climaxes fail because women get distracted by worrying about the children, or the neighbours banging on the wall, or the thought of being late for work. One woman gave me the following wonderful description of misery:

> You can love any man in the world, but you can't make love to a man with a mobile phone. It just doesn't work. You've got him all relaxed and your hands are gliding into each other's knickers when 'ring, ring'. OK, so business is business. The world can't wait just because you're dying for a screw. That settled, you strip off his trousers and he goes down on his knees and unzips yours and begins . . . 'ring, ring'. Hell, you think, the world can't be that desperate, but it is, and you wait, and then he drags you to the floor and fits in nice and gently and begins to move real slow.

'Ring, ring.'
And so it goes on. Forget it. You might as well fuck a
telephone box.

These are obvious distractions. But are you aware of just how
distracting *local* elements can be? Elements that you'd always
thought of as part and parcel of your lovemaking. The need to
return his kisses, to keep fondling his penis, to answer his sweet
nothings, to indicate your responsiveness when he fondles you. Of
course these things *are* important; one doesn't do it merely because
of need, but because one wants to return kisses, to fondle and
exchange murmurs of devotion and delight. Sex is emotional, not
a cold race for orgasm. Furthermore, these pleasant 'distractions'
help to create the mood, to make us feel aroused. All this is true,
but the fact remains that for the woman inexperienced in coital
orgasm these 'distractions' can be disruptive.

To return to the foreign language analogy – it's work for a
United Nations interpreter, listening and translating *at the same
time*, not a job for a fairly new Teach Yourself student, who still
needs a bit of practice. When you first start to learn a language or
to have an orgasm you have to think very hard and concentrate on
what you're doing. Later, when you're fluent, it comes more
readily, often without thinking at all. I'm not saying you should
strip away these 'distractions' altogether, but I am saying that
while you are training yourself you should sometimes try to
suspend them. You'll be able to return them tenfold if, later, you
don't have the worry of orgasm to bother you.

Next time you make love I want you to relax and as far as
possible *forget all about your surroundings*. If necessary even try to
forget about *him*. Close your eyes and concentrate on one thing:
what he is doing to you, the movement of his buttocks, his penis
sliding in and out. Or choose a favourite fantasy and concentrate
on that. Ruth's worked well, but she also had reservations about
it:

I like to think I'm on a small island, lying on the beach
taming one of the natives between my thighs. But I wonder

> if it would be better if I concentrated on the fact that I'm
> really on the floor with my boyfriend Harry? Surely
> fantasy detracts from concentration and therefore from
> orgasm?

Fantasy does not detract from orgasm if used correctly; it is an
extremely important *aspect of concentration*. The fantasy acts as a
stimulating focus for your concentration. The thing that matters
now is *your sexual needs*, not the natives, or your boyfriend. Therefore
use whichever *works*.

At this stage don't worry about pleasing him: if you are busy
nuzzling his ear, or showing what a skilful lover you are by tickling
his balls and sucking on his tongue, chances are your concentration
is draining away. Besides, the last thing you want just now is to
help him any closer to *his* orgasm.

Juliet also had reservations about concentrating too much on
her own pleasure:

> I've got a fairly new boyfriend and I feel I have to show
> him some attention and appreciation while we make love,
> or he'll think me unfeeling. And I couldn't possibly *tell*
> him what to do.

Of course you must show some attention and appreciation in a
new relationship. The idea is simply not to let this get in the way
of your own training. The trick is to make telling him *what* to do
part and parcel of telling him that you like what he is doing. For a
start, we've seen that men dislike unresponsive women. But there
are two ways of being responsive. You can either say baldly, 'I
love what you're doing,' or you can *imply* by encouraging him to
continue with a certain thing: 'Mmmmm, do this, no – like this,
yes, mmmm. Please go on.' The second – if you think carefully
about it – is a far more seductive way of saying that you like his
attentions. In fact the more deeply involved you are in enjoying his
attentions – and therefore the more distracted in praising them –
the more profound is your appreciation. As long as you are loving
and attentive some of the time, you need have no fear that during

that crucial lead up to orgasm you are quiet and concentrated. And the thought of mutual pleasure should be far more satisfying to him than a couple of lost last-minute kisses.

Exercise 10.2 Here is a tip I have found extremely helpful. One of the women who had used this programme suggested to me the following:

> For some reason – I can't explain why – when I'm very worked up, I clench my vagina tightly. If I keep that up for quite a few minutes it really gives me a big boost towards orgasm.

This may remind you of the Kegel exercises I discussed in Chapter 5 (which, by the way, you should be still practising). The vaginal muscles developed by those exercises – the P-C or pubococcygeal muscles – are the same ones you should try tensing in this exercise.

Tensing your muscles is a well known way of increasing arousal. You may find that clenching other muscles, such as your stomach, legs, feet and hands, makes you feel closer to orgasm. Conversely, for men, an ancient technique of helping to delay orgasm is relaxing all the muscles, especially in the legs and bottom.

THE DISEMBODIED WOMAN

Discussing concentration leads naturally on to a phenomenon I have called the Disembodied Woman. It is an aspect of sex that is rarely – if ever – recognized in sex manuals. Yet it can be crucial to your success.

When you have sex with your partner, many things come into play. Not only is he thrusting his penis in and out of you, he may also be stimulating your breasts, nuzzling your earlobe, etc. The point is that these things can detract from your orgasm *even when they increase your overall desire.*

Obviously if you don't enjoy him stimulating your breasts, it risks detracting from your ability to climax. But for many women, even when it *heightens* their overall excitement, it can still lead them down the wrong path – the path *away* from orgasm. The reason is because it replaces that badly needed concentration on orgasm with a more diffuse sensual pleasure. Now this more diffuse pleasure is all very well, but if you're feeling a little dodgy about orgasm, it can tip the balance in your disfavour. As Sally explains, it's almost as if for some women (some of the time, at least) there are

> two parts to me. On the one hand there's the orgasm. I may want to have one very much or I mightn't mind too badly, but whatever my desire for it I must either go full out for it alone or give it up. I've got to get the timing right and the rhythm and so on. I've got to think only about the feeling in my groin. It's like coming up to a hurdle in the steeplechase: you've got to make sure you jump from the right foot at the right time with the right stride and so on. On the other hand, there are the general body pleasures. I can just lie back and enjoy the idea of sex, or the feel of his hand playing over me, or the intimacy of his kissing and affections – but if I do that I'm limiting my chances of coming. As if my friends who'd come to watch me jump the hurdle began an interesting conversation amongst themselves as I ran towards it.

Now you may well not be this sort of woman. If you are, you must learn to distinguish those aspects of your lovemaking that directly contribute to orgasm, and those that, however pleasant in themselves, can prove distractions. I have little hesitation in saying that, once you become more adept at it, these distinctions will matter very much less – if at all.

Try the following:

Exercise 10.3 Start making love with your partner. Begin with the usual methods that get you aroused. These may include stroking your thighs, kissing your breasts, biting your neck – whatever. But as you become extremely aroused, get your partner to stop these attentions and concentrate only on the actual act of penetration or of clitoral stimulation. Do you feel yourself getting closer to orgasm, or further away?

A WORD ABOUT LUBRICATION

All the sex manuals tell you that when women get sexually excited their vaginas become naturally lubricated. As one put it, lubrication is the equivalent of the erection – a physical manifestation of sexual arousal. What they usually omit to say is that not all women do this, and that that is quite normal too. However excited I am feeling I rarely have enough lubrication when we begin.

For a long time I hid this, ashamed of yet another 'failure'. After all, the randy woman with her 'dripping cunt' is the crude byword of sexual arousal. In fact it is quite usual for a woman not to get lubricated – from nervousness, change in hormones, or simply because she's made that way.

All you have to do is use some other sort of lubrication. KY Jelly – available at the chemist – is a colourless jelly which you would really need to apply before you begin. But for those women who need only a little warming up before they get wet, I personally think there is nothing better than saliva: it does the job well and it's readily available. No getting up to go to the bathroom, and no nastiness if you go on to oral sex. Apply a large amount to your first two fingers and smear it up *inside* and around the entrance to your vagina. This has the great advantage that it can be done surreptitiously while lying down before he puts his penis in. Alternatively, the man can provide the lubrication on his own penis. For Barbara, the act of lubricating is an important part of lovemaking.

My favourite moment is when David straddles me. I always prop my pillows up so I can see him lick his hands, then slowly take his own dick and rub the saliva all over it. There's something very sexy about a guy rubbing his own dick. And something slightly threatening, in the nicest way possible, about seeing him preparing himself to fuck you.

SEXUAL TIMING: HIS VERSUS YOURS

One of the biggest problems a woman has to contend with is that she will almost certainly take longer to reach orgasm than the man. 'Surely one of Nature's great practical jokes,' said one male friend, 'only not a very funny one. Men have orgasms quickly and then it's all over, while women want to do it slowly, and usually more than once.'

Mind you, the hasty lover is in distinguished company if this limerick by Norman Douglas is anything to go by:

> There was a young lady of Thun,
> Who was blocked by the Man in the Moon,
>   'Well, it has been great fun,'
>   She remarked when he'd done,
> 'But I'm sorry you came quite so soon.'

Man in the Moon or no, a good lover should be able to control his orgasm; but then a good lover is not always to hand. Remember that, ideally, you should *both* be learning at the same time. *You* are learning to have an orgasm, while *he* is learning *not* to have his too soon. (You might remind him that a man known to have staying power is *always* in demand.)

On the whole young men are more prone to ejaculating too soon – but they have the great advantage that they can get another erection again very quickly. And, as Juliet found out, some young men can do even better than that:

He was spending the summer vacation before going up to university in a farmhouse I owned, studying. He was really diligent, but nice, polite and not bad looking. He invited me up to his room for supper once, and one thing led to another and I seduced him before we got to the dessert. He was really nervous (which got me going something terrible) and began making excuses, saying things like he didn't have a condom, but I told him to be quiet. I could tell he wanted me. I got him quickly on to the bed (the only time I ever regretted giving my tenant a cheap mattress!) and we did it for about an hour, non-stop, and he didn't come once. I was crushed. I thought: I made a mistake. He didn't fancy me, he only did it because I owned the place. I felt ugly and unattractive. Two hours later I found out he'd ejaculated twice and still gone on – but had been shy and controlled enough to prevent me noticing, because he thought he'd been too quick. We're still together.

The major problem with the woman taking a long time is that it causes anxiety, which hinders orgasm. This was constantly happening to me in the early stages. I could have done it reasonably soon if only I hadn't been worrying that I was taking too long: a vicious circle.

The most common means to get round such a problem is by having a lot of foreplay. I'd teach my partner how to rub me gently, and then make him do it until I was worked up to a pitch. But this carries a drawback: even when I had a nice bloke who said he didn't mind, and would wait, particularly since he liked it lasting a long time, I felt guilty that he was having to please me and so was prevented from pleasing himself. Another vicious circle. In time, you can get used to this, and overcome the feeling of tension. But it's often a good idea to have a couple of occasions when he really is slowed down. So, if necessary, you must revert to any subterfuge that will put you at ease – as Esther does:

If I know I'm going to want it in the evening, I give him a blow job in the day. Just after he gets back from work.

This slows him down later in the evening and makes him feel he owes me something, too.

Alternatively, if you've done it before going to sleep, wake him up again in the night. Remember also that tired and tipsy men do it more slowly. So many women tend to write off a man who looks blotto, exhausted or pickled. This is a wicked waste. Instead, as I've suggested before, be inventive in using these occasions. They can be wonderfully helpful in defusing a potential argument, or in avoiding that threatening, macho style of sex.

As a very last resort, ask a Fairy Godmother to turn you both into minks. Those darling little animals have been known to spend as much as eight hours in intercourse. It gives a whole new meaning to why women are supposed to yearn for a mink coat.

MAKING USE OF A LIMP PENIS

You may be lucky and have a man who is willing – and able – to go on. But if the worst comes to the worst, don't despair. Although we have all been taught to think of an erect penis as necessary for a woman's satisfaction, this is not true at all. If your man ejaculates, it is not a disaster. Encourage him to leave his penis in position – which, sleepy and satisfied, he may be very happy to do. Simply continue to rub yourself as you have learned to do in step 4. Some penises remain hard for a long time afterwards, others go limp very quickly. Whichever is the case you can use it to your advantage. Sandra takes up the theme:

> I was full of the usual prejudices when I met Peter: a big stiff cock was what was needed to satisfy a woman, and as I had never had an orgasm, when I first saw Peter's my hopes soared. I had fucked a dozen men, and had always had a sense of being close to climaxing, but never actually getting there. One day we started fucking in the middle of the afternoon. I'd been looking forward to a long, slow

session, and I was furious when he came after just ten minutes. My first thought was to go to the bathroom and masturbate – my usual way of getting satisfaction. But he fell asleep and somehow I hadn't the heart to just push him off. That was my liberation.

I began to rub myself, with his cock still inside me. I found that with him half asleep I could really relax and enjoy it. After a while his cock started getting a bit limp, but for some reason it felt not less satisfying but more. It was as if it was less of a threat, less aggressive, more soft and gentle and responsive. I don't think I'd ever enjoyed sex so much up until that moment – suddenly I found I was having a strong orgasm, round his penis.

That was a turning point for me. I realized I could do it with a man. Up until then I'd had a sort of mental block, thinking I'd never be able to. The next day I encouraged him to do the same. When he wanted to roll off me I said No, no, please stay there, I like to feel you. I practised every day – and three weeks later I had my first orgasm with him actually fucking me. I know it would never have happened but for that first time. He doesn't know that it was his limp prick that started me off – perhaps one day I'll tell him. He's quite macho about that sort of thing. I'd like to see his face!

Sandra made use of a penis that had gone limp inside her. It is also possible to get pleasure from one that has not gone hard at all. If your partner is unable to get an erection, don't reject him. With a little ingenuity (and his consent, of course) you can manipulate even a limp penis inside you. It'll probably have to be the Missionary Position; then once it's in, he makes gentle, rather minimal thrusting movements with his hips. Obviously it's not the same as sex with a sonking great erection – in many ways it's more pleasant: less threatening, and there is more concentration on your clitoral area.

I strongly suggest you give it a try. But make sure your attitude is that this is something pleasant *in itself*, not a second best because he can't get a hard-on. That way you are doing his confidence a great deal of good and, almost certainly, helping him to overcome his erection problems.

HOW TO DEAL WITH PREMATURE EJACULATION

Women whose partners suffer from premature ejaculation – that is, not just sloppy lovemaking but genuine inability to prevent themselves coming almost before you've begun – have both advantages and disadvantages.

The disadvantages are obvious: little or no penetration. Like difficulty with orgasm for women, premature ejaculation is the most common male sexual complaint. Both can be readily cured by training.

The advantage of a premature ejaculator for the woman on this programme is not simply that he owes you plenty of attention – but that *he knows he owes it to you*. It was probably nervous bluff anyway. Premature ejaculation can be very distressing for the man who suffers from it, so it goes without saying that you must be kind. But then, because you understand sexual difficulties, you probably *will* be kind. Mutual sympathy for each other's problems can greatly strengthen a relationship. You may even find that you'd both like to try going to a sex therapist. It is in this area that they have the most success. But if you do, don't give up this programme, just adapt it to your circumstances. Outside help can be extremely useful, but it rarely beats self-training. So, even though premature ejaculation will delay your training for this step, don't worry – be inventive, not defeatist.

Make sure there is foreplay *and* afterplay. Teach him how to use his hands and mouth. Concentrate on side-steps A (manual) and B (oral). If you can learn to climax under these circumstances, the chances are you will find it a small step to climaxing with a penis once his premature ejaculation is cured.

And just to show that not all women want a man to spin it out, let me quote you another Norman Douglas limerick:

> There was a young lady of Kew,
> Who said, as the curate withdrew:
>   'I prefer the dear vicar;
>   He's longer and thicker;
> Besides, he comes quicker than you.'

CHAPTER ELEVEN

STEP 6: SUCCESS AND HOW TO BUILD ON IT

Congratulations! By now you've probably had your first *trained* orgasm with your lover. The hard work is behind you. Now it is only a matter of practice and expanding your abilities.

KEEP IMPROVING

Before I had my first orgasm I used to think that women were divided into two categories: those who could have orgasms and those who could not. That when you'd done it once there would be no more problems and you would do it ever after. If only! The truth is very much more complex than that, as those readers who began this book having experienced only occasional orgasms will know. Now you must build on your ability gradually.

So here it is in capitals, the Golden Rule:

KEEP PRACTISING AT ALL LEVELS

And this means:

1. Keep improving your masturbation techniques.
2. Keep finding times to have sex where there is no question of it ending in orgasm.
3. Keep having sex and orgasm occasionally without penetration.

Your first *self-trained* orgasm is a sexual milestone. For those who've never done it before it represents positive proof that things can get better. You will never look back. What you are going to aim for now is an orgasm each time you want one, with the minimum of effort – and eventually several orgasms if you and your partner feel like it. From now on they will gradually get more and more frequent. More importantly, they will cease to be a hit-and-miss affair. Even on the days when you don't come, you will understand why it is and what went wrong.

WHAT ABOUT WHEN I DON'T CLIMAX?

Unless you are a very remarkable woman indeed, there will always be the odd day when you don't climax: because you're feeling anxious, or painful, or simply off-colour, or you may have had too much to drink – there are all sorts of reasons. Don't worry about these days. With practice and repetition of the exercises, they will become fewer. Besides, I can pretty much guarantee that once you know you *can* do it, you will no longer be distressed when you don't. The whole subject of orgasm, which assumed such gigantic proportions when you couldn't do it, now seems just one pleasant aspect of life.

In the early days of your success, however, you may still feel impatient to climax and be disappointed when you don't. On these occasions instead of sighing in despair *take action*. Get out your pen and paper and analyse what went wrong. Some of the possible causes of failure are:

1. Local circumstances wrong – light on, felt nervous, people walking about outside the bedroom door, etc.
2. Outside causes – drank too much, felt too sleepy, etc.
3. Lousy lover – perhaps he came too soon, or neglected to give you any attention.
4. I simply didn't fancy my partner.

All this is still part of the process of gaining control and mastery over your own body and lovemaking. You will get more and more adept at knowing what circumstances upset your skill, and you will learn either to cope with them or to avoid them altogether.

HOW TO MEASURE YOUR SUCCESS

It's always helpful to chart your successful achievements. The language student will be taking exams – you have other means. I measured my success at orgasm in three ways:

1. By *how often* I could do it. At first, as you know, I couldn't do it at all. Gradually training brought it up to approximately one orgasm every three times I made love. Now I do so every time I want to, sometimes two or three times a night.

2. By *how readily* I could do it, regardless of non-ideal circumstances. For example, I used to find orgasm impossible if I'd been drinking, or if I felt tense after a hard day at the office. Now these factors make very little difference.

3. By my *versatility* – different positions, different places in the house, etc. This really is the fun part. As you build up your repertoire, you will become more adventurous. You will learn to do it standing up, or out in the open. The more versatile you are, the more your confidence will grow, and that in turn will help your ability to reach orgasm.

Obviously the rate of your progress will depend to some extent upon the quality of your lover – even more so in the early stages. If necessary sit him down and train him, too. *All* men need instruction in sex, and very few get it. Most importantly, get him to read Chapter 18 of this book, which has been written specially for him. If you want to keep the rest of the book secret, photocopy those pages and tell him a friend at work passed it on to you.

THE INTENSITY OF YOUR ORGASM

Just as in masturbation, you will find that the intensity of your orgasms with a partner varies a great deal. Some days they may be strong, other days weak. I've never found any real reason why some orgasms explode while others just fizzle, although a friend of mine made the following curious connection:

> I've noticed that if I'm *really* randy – you know, aching for it – my orgasm is a great relief but not necessarily top quality. Yet several times when I haven't been thinking of sex at all, and Jeff's come along and persuaded me, it takes a while to get me going but when I do climax it's incredibly intense.

Other women, like Melanie, claim that it depends on their state of mind, physical comfort, or even the sex position they adopt:

> If I had to think of a pattern I suppose it's that the best orgasms are the most easygoing ones, when I'm not think-ing to myself, 'Oh, God, when will I come?' and so on. It depends on position too of course. Oral sex, particularly the way Mark does it – I don't know where he learnt it from but I hope it was a book and not one of those fancy tarts – just collapses me. Missionary is usually never quite so strong.

Just keep up the good work, and the good results will follow.

Masters and Johnson concluded from their researches that the most intense orgasms came not from intercourse with a man, but from masturbation. You won't be surprised to learn, academics being what they are, that other researchers disagree. What do *you* think? You are now in a position to answer that question yourself.

SIMULTANEOUS ORGASM

Now here's a subject that causes a lot of squabbling. Many writers talk of the beauty of simultaneous orgasm with your partner. Personally I think it's greatly overrated. It is, of course, a standard requirement of lovers in romantic fiction. Perhaps the most ludicrous description I've come across is 'twin internal explosions'. D.H. Lawrence's famous erotic novel *Lady Chatterley's Lover* also expresses the ideal of climaxing together, and the likes of Frank Harris would not be complete without a good mutual orgasm:

> 'Let me,' I cried, and, in a moment, I was on her, working my organ up and down on her clitoris, the porch, so to speak, of Love's temple. A little later she herself sucked the head into her hot, dry pussy and then closed her legs as if in pain to stop me going further; but I began to rub my sex up and down on her tickler, letting it slide right in every now and then, till she panted and her love-juice came and my weapon sheathed itself in her naturally. I soon began the very slow and gentle in-and-out movements which increased her excitement steadily while giving her more and more pleasure, till I came and immediately she lifted my chest up from her breasts with both hands and showed me her glowing face. 'Stop, boy,' she gasped, 'please, my heart's fluttering so! I came too, you know, just with you,' and indeed I felt her trembling all over convulsively.

All very dandy to read about, but is it what we should be aiming for?

I don't think so. Simultaneous orgasm is nice (all orgasms are nice), but it's not necessarily the high point of good sex. The fuss made over it is largely because film directors, pulp fiction writers and some sexually distressed geniuses have adolescent fantasies about the matter.

I view simultaneous orgasm with great caution. It's relatively easy for a man to choose the moment when he ejaculates – at least if he puts his mind to it – but it's extremely difficult for most women to do so. And who gets the blame when it goes wrong? You've guessed it.

In fact, simultaneous orgasm has some serious drawbacks. First, and perhaps most important from the point of view of women on this plan, worrying about timing is the last thing you need. You'd do far better to establish with your partner that you have *no* intention of trying to come at the same time he does. I take great care to make sure my partner understands this at the beginning of any new relationship. If he wants us to come together, then *he* must time his orgasm, not I mine – it's much easier for him than it is for me. Another disadvantage of simultaneous orgasm is that if you work too hard to have it, then you'll often find your own climax to be diminished as a result.

But perhaps most importantly, to my mind, it's a serious impediment to one of the greatest pleasures of all – savouring your partner's orgasm – because you're far too busy being carried away by your own. And, what's more, you also risk losing much of the pleasure of your partner's exciting *build up* to orgasm, because you are too preoccupied with getting your own to work on cue.

For Sally, the greatest drawback of simultaneous orgasm is that

> it doesn't allow the enormous pleasure of having Mike go on after I've climaxed. If I come first then there's nothing sexier than to feel his penis moving inside of me in time to my contractions and then a little later to watch him gasp with the same pleasure that I've just enjoyed.

To expand on Sally's comment briefly, many women have stated that one of the most enjoyable sensations is to let the man continue thrusting after they've climaxed. Writes Leslie:

> I very rarely climax twice, but after I've had my orgasm I feel wonderfully liberated. I no longer have the anxiety of

making sure I come before he does, and my orgasm leaves me feeling terribly responsive. Those five or so minutes between my orgasm and his are the best. And there's always the hope that you *might* do it twice, after all.

So my advice is: *don't* view simultaneous orgasm as something to aim for. If it happens, let it happen naturally.

MULTIPLE ORGASM

Multiple orgasms are, famously, an almost exclusively female talent. Even with men who can come more than once in a row, there's usually a limp period after the first ejaculation. Naturally, this inequality has given rise to a lot of extravagant fantasy and prejudice. Some men have dreams about satisfying the insatiable woman (Frank Harris, once again, and dozens of other writers of similar 'confessions'). Others – the Roman satirist Juvenal was a particularly bad case – prefer simply to grouse about women being naturally insane with lust. In both cases, of course, such attitudes say more about the men who hold them than the women they have in mind. Sometimes you'll even come across stories in which the woman has all her orgasms during the time that the man is having his one.

'When I was a boy,' a friend wrote to me recently,

I used to dread the idea of going to bed with a woman. Absolutely awful. I thought all you had to do was touch one in the wrong place and she'd start going off like a jackhammer. And I'd heard that women liked to claw your back and scream at the top of their voices during sex. I couldn't figure out why anyone would want to go through with it.

Outside of the usual nonsense, there's been a lot of serious interest in women's ability to have more than one orgasm, but not many conclusions. True multiple orgasms, that is several orgasms with no or hardly any break in between, are a luxury and very rare. I've certainly never had them. 'Sequential' is one orgasm after another with pauses to cool down in between. Sequential orgasms are much more common and certainly within the reach of many women. I've already stated that in masturbation one can quickly improve one's personal best. The same is true of orgasms with a partner, except that progress is a little slower.

Some women find they feel too sensitive to be touched after the first orgasm, but those who boldly continue often report subsequent orgasms increasing in intensity.

The biggest barrier to more than one orgasm per session is often the attitudes of the women themselves, who feel 'greedy', 'unnatural' or 'a nymphomaniac' for having more than their partner. If this is your problem, try looking at it this way: if men and women ought to have an equal amount of sexual pleasure, without one or the other being 'greedy', let's reckon it out over a lifetime. That way you've got an awful lot of catching up to do.

SOLO ORGASM

Now here's some advice that is seldom put forward. What I call 'solo orgasm' is when one partner brings the other to a climax, without taking anything in return. Rosalind explains:

> I was sitting at my desk at home, going through the bills one Saturday afternoon. Bob came in. He took hold of me and led me to the bedroom. On the bed he stripped off my skirt, my panties and threw open my legs. Then for half an hour he just concentrated on giving me oral sex. I protested a bit at first – but, what the devil, it felt great!
>
> He kept on at me with his tongue till I came – twice, as a matter of fact, which is unusual. Then he simply stood up and walked off, leaving me collapsed on the bed and the bills still unpaid . . . I thought I was seeing things at

first – I mean men normally want something in return. But he said No, he'd take his dues later. It's something we do quite often now; we both find it extraordinarily sexy.

Solo orgasm is, of course, particularly helpful for the woman on this programme because she has no distractions whatsoever. We are all familiar with the old scenario of the man who demands or begs for a 'blow job' or 'a bit of manual relief' – and bloody irritating it can be. But if you can engineer a situation where you *both* do it to each other, at different times, that's great. It's easy enough for you to sidle up to him – but you'll need a sensitive and understanding partner to do the same back.

Get into the habit of solo sex. Mutual pleasure is great too, but selfishness is a delight once in a while.

THE UNPALATABLE MALE

I want now to take a look at some of the more intangible problems you may be faced with.

Fear of the penis, and all it represents, is a common one – more common than you may think. However much we feel aroused, there is no doubt that a naked man, with a 7-inch erect penis, can be threatening. As Juliet points out:

It's not so much that it looks large because I like the idea of a big one, but that it looks so bloody uncompromising. Once you see it you can't help thinking 'goodbye tenderness, hello beast'. Some days I don't mind so much, but it can seem such an unemotional thing.

This sort of abstract anxiety is at the heart of a lot of female sexual dissatisfaction. For Pat it was plain old distaste:

Such a big, red, horrid-looking object. I can't remember where it was, but I remember reading as a child in some

dirty book (it might have been a copy of De Sade that my
father kept in the liquor cabinet) about the penis's purple
head and red balls. A cock was always painted in the most
lurid colours. I was quite curious about it at the time,
although my brother's example proved a little disappointing. But later, when I saw one properly while cramped in
the back of a car after a date with a college boy, I almost
felt sick. I mean all those veins and that sort of 'throbbing'
look. It looked like a growth, a tumour maybe. So ugly.

Both of these responses – fear and distaste – are well known.
Some women feel them frequently or all the time, most feel them
occasionally to varying degrees. These feelings are not to be
dismissed. Recognize and acknowledge them, then take steps.
Below is a short list of suggestions I've received from women: some
of them are more light-hearted than others, but I'm assured they
all work.

1. Explore him all over while he's lying down, after you've made
love: it's important that you grow familiar with his body in
circumstances that aren't about to become purely sexual. If you
can arrange it with him, lay off full sex for a while, and instead
spend the time exploring each other's bodies and talking to each
other about how you feel. If need be, get him to masturbate just
before in private, so that when you are together his penis is not
erect and there's no suggestion that sex is to follow. After a few
sessions like this get him to masturbate in your presence and then
play gently but undemandingly with each other afterwards. By
progressing in this manner, slowly becoming more familiar with
the penis as a non-aggressive, sensitive object of pleasure, you will
gradually build up confidence and lower your fear or distaste.

2. Let his penis go limp inside you: after he's ejaculated, make
him stay put until you feel it slip right out of you. The importance
of this suggestion is in allowing you to appreciate both the strengths
and weaknesses of the penis and the male sex drive.

3. Watch his penis grow small after sex: hold it gently after
ejaculation and withdrawal. The more you familiarize yourself
with the whole process the better your understanding and the less

your unease. I find that just after ejaculation, when it is half up and half down, the penis is at its best.

4. Hold the erect penis in your hand, moisten the head and rub it gently around your mouth, just as if you were applying lipstick. This is a lovely exercise, because the head is the softest, gentlest part.

5. If he's a great big stud of a man whom you met at the party the night before, *catch him in his underpants and socks*. That'll bring him down to size.

6. Think of as many words for 'penis' as you can. Some of them are so delightful or ridiculous – Percy Plonker, for example – that one ends up feeling quite affectionate towards the dear little things.

7. Say the word 'penis' itself ten times: you'll realize what a comic word it is. Keep saying it and you'll soon be laughing out loud. The woman who recommended this invented a wonderful, silly game that had her and her friends all rolling in the aisles. She found some popular songs and substituted 'penis' for one of the main words of the song, which they then all sang aloud, with much wine flowing. The favourite was 'How Much Is That Penis In The Window?'.

CHAPTER TWELVE

SIDE-STEP A: MANUAL SEX

The great advantage of the man arousing the woman by manual sex is that it can be done almost anywhere: in the cinema, driving a car, at a party, standing in a queue – the possibilities are endless, and the variations infinite. One friend of mine used to get his girlfriend to climax during the rush hour on the tube, while the two of them were standing, strap-hanging, pressed closely together. It can be done with your clothes on or off, in private or in public, with penetration (of your partner's fingers) or without, as foreplay or afterplay . . .

So why does manual sex come as a side-step in the programme, rather than as a logical progression from masturbation?

The answer is partly because many people still regard manual sex as not quite respectable, and partly because men are notoriously bad at using their hands.

It's not entirely men's fault. Manual sex on a woman is a very difficult thing to do well. On a man it is relatively easy – the penis is a large and well-defined organ, which needs a certain amount of fairly vigorous, unimaginative attention. There are extra tricks that a woman can learn – sex manuals are always going on about them – but the great majority of men seem perfectly happy with the basic rub-a-dub-dub.

A woman, however, has a very delicate, sophisticated sexual area. What's more, women vary from individual to individual in what they find most stimulating. As one female friend of mine put

153

it, 'I'm damned glad I don't have to make love to another woman. I wouldn't have the first clue about how to arouse her, or where to fiddle!' The anonymous *A Protest by the Medical Profession* contains the following verse:

There's the vulva, the vagina and the jolly perineum;
There's the hymen which is sometimes found in brides;
There's the uterus, the clitoris, the ovum and the oviducts,
The ovaries and Lord knows what besides.

It's no surprise, then, that men, whose sexual experience with their hands is normally limited to masturbation, are usually a little cack-handed when it comes to satisfying a woman's needs manually.

The trouble is not enough men have the tact – or the courage – to ask which technique their partner likes. Too many either consider it a slight to their manhood to hesitate and show ignorance, or fear that the woman will mock him as being inadequate. This seems to me one of the great tragedies of relations between the sexes. Because for most women the idea of a man who bothers to ask what she likes is a dream come true, not a cause for mockery. However, until communication between men and women improves, this miserable misunderstanding will continue. Let me simply repeat – for the benefit of any stray male reader – *there is no reason why men should feel shy or small in admitting that they don't know their way about down there*. Joline, usually rather a reticent woman, becomes quite outspoken and lyrical on the subject.

I always say that there are two aspects to a good lover – his hands and his questions. If he uses his hands sensitively, exploring and investigating, never crude but always responsive, then he's got the makings of a prince of pleasure. He should ask questions with his hands as well as his mouth. His hands should notice what gestures are effective, what rhythm most pleasing, and his mouth should be ready to ask verbally if the sexual signs are too difficult for him to interpret.

It is, in short, ignorance and lack of communication which often makes manual sex more difficult for women than it ought to be. That is why I've put it in as a side-step. Personally, I only succeeded after progressing through steps 1–4, largely because my partner at the time – a nice guy, I'm still in touch with him – had hands that reminded me of a trouser press. Other women, however, have succeeded at an earlier stage of the programme. It's up to you when you try it. And remember, whatever the standard of your lover, with a little bit of ingenuity you can usually improve the situation a good deal.

MANUAL SEX WITH CLOTHES ON

Begin your manual sex programme with your clothes on. I want you and your lover to try to do each exercise successfully three times before you can really feel you have mastered it. You may either stick to the same exercise until you achieve this, or you may alternate with another exercise. Do not, however, attempt more than two types of exercise at any one time. After you have moved on, you should still repeat the previous exercises periodically.

The concentration will be on you, so you must decide whether or not to see to your partner's needs beforehand or afterwards (assuming you do so at all, that is). Men who haven't yet been satisfied sometimes get impatient for their turn, which will inhibit you. On the other hand, some women prefer to satisfy their lover afterwards because they have a partner who, once satisfied, tends to lose interest altogether. Only you can decide.

A very good friend of mine found herself in a situation similar to that described by Erica Jong in *Fear of Flying* (quoted in Chapter 15). She was crossing Europe by train, but in a completely full carriage. As none of the passengers had paid for a sleeper, when night fell a guard brought round blankets which everybody snuggled into sitting upright. Somehow my friend found herself pleasantly and secretly beneath the blanket exchanging manual sex with the young man sitting next to her. 'Heavenly,' she concluded. 'I never even learned his name.'

Exercise 12.1 To begin arrange situations in which your lover arouses you with your clothes on, when it's acknowledged by both of you *before you begin* that you're not aiming for full orgasm. Arrange the situation so that it enforces this restraint (re-read step 3 for advice).

Do this exercise in circumstances you find most relaxing and suitable, but don't do it in the bedroom. I want you to avoid the undesirable orgasm-as-goal situation.

Exercise 12.2 As above, but vary the circumstances. Wear different clothes; do it at different times, in unusual settings. But, once more, avoid the bedroom. If you are sitting in the cinema there is no danger that he is going to try to go too far. A little gentle rubbing while watching the film can be a very constructive thing. You can relax completely because *nothing depends on it*. All in all try to make it a normal part of your relationship that he gives you manual stimulation now and then when you're out together for whatever purpose.

Re-read step 2 on masturbation for a further discussion of the possibilities. Masturbation and manual sex have numerous similarities and you can model your progression here on your masturbation progression.

By all means give him occasional attention and encouragement while he's doing it (some kisses, stroking his penis) but no more than that. This is *your* time, and you must feel free to concentrate.

Exercise 12.3 As above, but now leave the outcome – orgasm or no orgasm – open. Don't say 'this time I'll come', just allow for the possibility of it. Give yourself a bit more time. As before, try to avoid the bedroom, but make extra sure that you're not going to worry about the amount of time you're taking, or the fact that all the attention is on you.

If you find that you do not climax, don't fuss. You have plenty of time, and there are other things you can be getting on with in the programme meanwhile. Keep practising. You will succeed.

Pass on to the next exercise only when you feel comfortable with your response to this one.

Exercise 12.4 This exercise is not strictly speaking manual, but it's definitely sexy. Lie in bed naked beneath the bedclothes. Now have your partner, also naked (at least on his lower half) lie on top of you. You open your legs and he presses his penis against you, as if in the Missionary Position. The crucial difference is that, of course, the bedclothes are between you. But the effect is similar to that of manual sex. See if you can reach orgasm this way.

MANUAL SEX WITH CLOTHES OFF

There are various scenarios for disaster when it comes to a man trying to stimulate a woman by manual sex. Most of us know them from bitter experience:

The man who sticks his finger in all the way and nothing else. A familiar species. A young man, quite likely a student. I seem to recall he's usually a bit spotty, eager, and uses that revolting phrase 'finger fucking'. Perhaps not to you, but probably to his pals. He shoves it in and out a bit – basically he thinks a woman's vagina is just an inside-out penis: you rub his on the outside, he does yours on the inside. This is the technique of the complete novice: the man who has never read about women's sexual organs, and certainly never bothered, or had the chance to ask a woman about them. By virtue of his being 'male' he thinks that knowing what to do to a woman is an 'instinct'.

The man who concentrates on the one spot to the exclusion of all else. This character has done some reading, or he's overheard a conversation in the pub. Perhaps someone has whispered to him that the clitoris is 'the seat of a woman's desire', nudge, nudge, wink, wink. Well, all I can say is you're a lucky woman if he's got the wrong spot. Because as we all know the clitoris is an immensely delicate organ that needs the most gentle handling. There's a residents' park in Hampstead that, ever since I climbed into it over the railings one night with an early boyfriend, makes me wince when I pass it. Because underneath the chestnut tree, he demonstrated his agonizing skill!

The man who is like a bull in a china shop. The particular specimen I had dealings with was a quantity surveyor, used to rubbing his hands over piles of bricks, I suppose . . . This tends to be another failing that results from men not appreciating that males and females have very different sexual organs and sensitivities. So once again it's car polishing time.

No doubt you can think of a number of other types. So for the exercises that follow, if your lover has certain manual faults spend some time educating him to be otherwise.

Exercise 12.5 Direct manual sex (as opposed to the indirect of the first three exercises) is much the easiest when you do not have your clothes on. Don't, to begin with, let him do it to you underneath your clothes – this restricts his movement and makes it harder to apply the proper pressure in the right places. So take your bottoms off, and lie in bed.

Manual sex as performed in bed has, of course, two classic functions: as foreplay to stimulate you and prepare you for full sexual intercourse. And as 'afterplay' in the event of the man ejaculating too soon. Make use of this. If you need or want to, bring him to climax first. Then let him concentrate on you.

The first few times you may want to establish beforehand that orgasm is not the goal – all you want to do is enjoy the sensations and become familiar with them. If orgasm follows, then all well and good, but the important thing, as ever, is not to worry about it and upset your sense of ease.

Apart from the immediate pleasure it gives, manual sex serves an important role in this programme: it gets you accustomed, gradually, to a sexual situation where *somebody else* is in physical control. Because of this it is worth experimenting with it. It is also important that you do not neglect the gains made by your training. Make sure that you maintain and improve on your ability, and try to establish it as an acceptable part of your normal sex life, and an alternative to intercourse, rather than merely as something to happen either before or after.

If you still have trouble enjoying yourself with manual sex, set up a situation on the bed at home that is as close as possible to your own familiar masturbation sessions. Now, as he attends to you, lie back and imagine you're masturbating alone. If necessary, use your own hands as well as his.

CHAPTER THIRTEEN

SIDE-STEP B: ORAL SEX

Like manual sex, oral sex can be introduced into the programme at any time after step 2. When you decide to do it will depend on the quality of your lover, the type of relationship you have with him, and also on the degree of confidence you have in yourself. If you have completed step 2 then you are making wonderful progress and are well on the way to your goal; but you may still feel that oral sex is something of an exotic option, and that you'd prefer to consolidate your gains in the traditional way before attempting it. This is your decision. It is important that you do it when *you* feel ready.

I think oral sex can be wonderful. But not everybody agrees. This is the other reason that I have made it a side-step in the programme. It is not crucial to your progress. It is an added star if you do it, but if you don't it in no way detracts from the huge gold star studded with rubies and diamonds you get for completing the main programme. I advise you to attempt it; but if, despite my arguments in its favour, you still think it somewhat beyond the pale, don't worry. If, on the other hand, you have no worries about it, and are eager to get on and learn how to make it serve you to best advantage, then you can skip what follows and go directly to the next section, 'Stage One'.

Oral sex – 'cunnilingus' when the man does it to the woman, 'fellatio' when it's the other way round – engenders strong feelings. I was in my twenties when Dr David Reuben's book *Everything You*

Always Wanted to Know about Sex (but were Afraid to Ask), hit the headlines. The following piece of extravagant nonsense clammed me up for years:

> **By simultaneous cunnilingus and fellatio every possible sense is brought to a fever pitch and a mutual orgasm occurs rapidly unless the couple switches to a penis-vagina position. The most presumably undersexed man or woman will be brought to an explosive orgasm by using this technique, providing they are willing to do it.**

If I had it my way I'd send the author to the lions' den, and throw in some vipers for good measure. Oral sex can be extremely satisfying, but for few couples is it so glib and easy as Dr Reuben describes. It is simply absurd (and somewhat savouring of cheap pornography) to suggest that mutual orgasm will occur because of it.

'Simultaneous cunnilingus and fellatio' consists in the man and woman lying top to toe with each other – either side by side, or one on top and one underneath – and simultaneously stimulating the genitals (because of the unusual position it is also often known as '69'). But it can be extremely uncomfortable for the woman, and should *never* be tried by the beginner. The guaranteed 'explosive orgasm', rapid or otherwise, is one of the most outrageously wicked promises I have ever heard. But it took me nearly two decades to find out.

Of all the many sexual myths, the idea that even the most 'undersexed' women will succumb to oral sex is one of the worst. First, it's simply not true. Second, it assumes that one man's method of cunnilingus is as good as another's, which is nonsense. Men's ability and skills vary wildly. Finally, it makes the woman for whom orgasm has never been easy (such as myself at the time of reading that book) so terrified that she is going to fail even where the most frigid have supposedly succeeded, that she freezes up completely. Stephen Vizinczey's novel *In Praise of Older Women* is the story of Adras Vadja, a young man, and his sexual encounters with – guess what? – older women. In it, Vadja's thoughts about his mistress' dislike of cunnilingus is a tribute to his sexual sensitivity on precisely this point.

> **There would be very few sexual problems if they could all be ascribed to inhibitions, yet at first I took it for granted that Paola refused to consent to any unfamiliar love-play out of modesty. However, her violent resistance showed not shyness but fear. It leaped through the blue of her eyes and hung over her long white body – the fear of false hopes and deeper defeats.**

Paola, having failed to have an orgasm in a more 'normal' way, fears yet another failure.

At the other extreme from Dr Reuben are those who consider oral sex dirty or perverted. Many women feel uncomfortable receiving oral sex – even the most liberated have confessed to their closest friends that they cannot relax while it is happening.

There are many reasons for these feelings, ranging from the obvious physical fact that a woman's genitals involve a hole and various funny extra bits that need regular washing, to the more subtle influence of a puritanical upbringing or the trauma of an earlier sexual encounter. None of these is to be dismissed lightly. If, whatever the cause, you feel uncomfortable with the *idea* of cunnilingus, then you will feel uncomfortable during the *act* of it. This is why the self-analysis of Stage One, below, is so important, even though it involves no physical contact.

STAGE ONE

It is of paramount importance that you get your ideas, hopes and fears about oral sex into perspective. Doing so constitutes the first part of this side-step. It is *not* the short route to success. You must train yourself here as you have trained elsewhere. But it can be, given a good lover and proper training of your own sexuality, one of the delights of making love. The tongue is a gentle, soft and versatile part of a man's body; I have often felt that there is no better use for it. If you feel that there is something fundamentally dirty about the process, or fear that your partner feels that there is, then you can always make a point of washing just beforehand, and making sure that he has noticed the fact. You might find it helpful to have a shower or bath together and wash each other during it.

And here I'd like to introduce a piece of good news: most men like doing oral sex. Virtually all the men I've asked about it agree that it's extremely sexy. If you don't believe me, just take a look at *Hite* on men.

In my case, a lot of my reservations about oral sex had to do with disastrous early cunnilingus. My partners might have enjoyed doing it, but they weren't much good. Let's face it, most sexually active women have some pretty dismal oral sex scenarios to relate – grim or comic, depending on which way you look at it. I hardly know a woman who hasn't had a good giggle with her friends over men's oral catastrophies.

Here are a few typical scenarios, some of them abominably reminiscent of the manual sex disasters of the previous chapter:

1. Down he goes, very purposeful and direct. He has read that the clitoris is the seat of sexual feeling, and having found it he's not going to let his concentration be diverted. He's made the mistake of assuming the clitoris is just like a penis. A painful mistake: it is much more sensitive. A good lover will spend much more time around the clitoris stimulating it indirectly. Not so, oral sexer number one: Just keep this up, he thinks, mistaking your writhes of agony for intense pleasure, and you'll be having an orgasm in no time.

2. This man's been told he has a long tongue, and he also thinks that the vagina is the seat of all passion. He sticks his tongue in and out simulating a penis, pausing every ten times or so because his mouth is tired. You, of course, feel little. His stubble scrapes on you.

3. The man of method. He's cultivated a Latin appearance – open-necked shirt, medallion, foreign sports car, possibly even funny-coloured sheets (black maybe). He thinks of oral sex as just one of the many courses on the sexual menu, somewhere between the foreplay starter and the coital main course. All you can think of while he's busy down there is that you've got pudding, dessert, cheese and coffee still to go – with increasing foreboding you wonder what they will consist of.

4. Rather a sporty type, this one. He doesn't really want to do it (although he doesn't mind if you do it to him) but he feels he must, or he's responding to your complaints. This man is rather fastidious. The penis, he thinks, is a straightforward thing, little more than a large finger really. Who ever minded sucking a finger? But all that funny stuff on a woman is a different story. OK, so it doesn't squirt a mess all over the place when it climaxes, but still, it can't be said to be a thing of great beauty, can it?

5. At last a civilized man! Everything is going well. You've settled down, got yourself comfortable, and begun to concentrate on the delicious feeling spreading through your body. He's not rough, or painful; he's moving his tongue around nicely and taking care to find your rhythm – and then he ruins it all by looking up and meeting your eye. Oh, the embarrassment of it! You don't know him very well, so there's no intimacy there. You'd just begun to let go when he starts staring past your breasts (which are too large), over your double-chin, up your nose and into your eyes. What a time to be caught unawares. My sister's boyfriend even used to wink!

If your worries about oral sex are more deep-seated – not confined to unsuitable partners – then it will pay to examine them carefully. If you still feel ill at ease, leave this chapter. You can always come back later, after you've made further progress in the main body of the programme.

STAGE TWO

As with all other parts of the programme, make sure that you are feeling comfortable and relaxed. If necessary, make a display of the fact that you have just washed yourself thoroughly before beginning: this is important not so much for his sake, but because it will put *you* at ease about *his* reservations. Naturally if you have any discharge or an unpleasant smell, don't do oral sex, and don't let yourself be pressured into it. Your lover may have a fetish about dirty knickers (don't laugh, some men do) but unless you share his delight it's best to steer clear. In fact there are men who love oral sex even with a menstruating woman. I know I could never feel at ease in such a situation, however much he reassured me. Remember: *nothing* must spoil your sense of ease.

In general the first few times it is best to do oral sex with as much anonymity as possible. A dark room can be immensely comforting. If you like, get him to do it while you are still largely clothed, or hiding beneath the bedcovers. The first time Laura ever managed to climax with oral sex was with the lights out and with the added sense of privacy from pulling the duvet over herself from the hips up, even over her face.

That way I wasn't in any doubt that Mark couldn't see all those bits I knew could have been smaller and thinner and a better shape. I mean, I hate all this dieting nonsense, but I'm just as much a victim of it as anybody else. I just can't get down to it [oral sex] without feeling uncomfortable and tensing up so much that he might as well be licking a lamppost. But that night I just covered my top up completely, while leaving my legs free so that I could move them about easily . . . It was such a silly position – and yet I *did* relax totally. I just let myself go. Mark's never been difficult about time. We just kept on, and I didn't have to look at him or see his movements to make me worry that he might be getting tired or bored, I just lay back and thought about me!

However, to begin with, *don't think about having an orgasm.* This will come later. The important thing is to introduce yourself to the sensations of oral sex, and to teach yourself to feel at ease with it.

If you feel awkward or embarrassed, pour yourself a drink. Alcohol slightly inhibits the physical ability to climax, but the relaxing effect will counteract this. Besides, to begin with you shouldn't be bothering about actually climaxing. A warm bath also helps to loosen you up, and makes you smell nice. Only when you begin to feel relaxed with the fact of oral sex should you start to think about concentrating on orgasm.

Paola (in *In Praise of Older Women*), whose refusal to even contemplate the idea of oral sex is uncompromising, finally has her first orgasm during cunnilingus because Vadja has approached her when at her most relaxed and least inhibited:

> Late one Saturday morning, I was awakened by the heat. The sun was shining into my eyes through the curved window panes and gauzy white curtains, and the temperature in the room must have been at least ninety degrees. During the night we had kicked off the blanket and the top-sheet, and Paola was lying on her back with her legs drawn up, breathing without a sound. We never look so much at the mercy of our bodies, in the grip of our unconscious cells, as when we are asleep. With a loud heartbeat, I made up my mind that this time I would make or break us. Slowly I separated her limbs: a thief parting branches to steal his way into a garden and rest his head. Though her body remained motionless, by then Paola must have been awake, but pretended not to be; she remained in that dreamy state in which we try to escape responsibility for whatever happens, by disclaiming both victory and defeat beforehand. It may have been ten minutes or half an hour later (time had dissolved into a smell of pine) that Paola's belly began to contract and let up and, shaking, she finally delivered up her joy, that offspring not even transient lovers can do without. When her cup ran over she drew me up by my arms and I could at last enter her with a clear conscience.
>
> 'You look smug,' were her first words when she focused her critical blue eyes again.

If your lover is the sort who feels no sex is good without orgasm, and you are uncomfortable or preoccupied with this feeling of his, then fake it. But tell yourself right at the beginning that you are going to fake it, and not halfway through, after you've begun to panic about not having a proper one.

The other familiar problem with oral sex was discussed above, namely the quality of your lover. But bear in mind that the man who knows 'how to do it' is simply the man who gives you pleasure. A little guidance from you might be in order.

At all costs avoid '69' at this early stage – as I'm sure Julia would agree:

> When I was in my teens '69' was all the go. The boys at school used to whisper about it. I was so naive that one day I asked the maths teacher what it was. He was a very young man, a supply teacher who was only there for a week or two. He went very red and pretended he hadn't heard. It was an omen, however, because after I'd left school and gone to college I met up with him by accident in a café. We got on really well and before long were sleeping together. One day he said did I remember that time when I'd asked him about '69'. Yes, I said, and then a little while later he arranged the position. My God, what a disappointment! I mean, by then I'd got to think of it as automatic orgasm, a real bang, but it was just bloody awkward. At first he went on top of me. He was bony, and his prick nearly choked me. Then I went on top of him and I worried that I'd flatten him. Then we tried it side by side but his neck got tired and he kept rolling away . . .

Let Julia's story be a lesson. Believe me, no woman is going to learn to have an orgasm while she is grappling upside-down with a man's penis. You might as well go straight back to square one.

STAGE THREE

Only once you have accommodated yourself to the idea of having a man down there should you start to concentrate on the possibility of orgasm. The interesting thing about oral sex is that when you *do* succeed it can be extremely intense – more intensely pleasurable than anything else.

Perhaps the most alluring description of oral sex comes from Katherine, who after many years of inability to climax in this way, now believes she's found the ultimate pleasure:

> I lie naked on my back while Freddy gives me oral sex. He makes it last a long time. He's naked too. Then, just as I feel myself beginning to climax – that wonderful point of no return – he moves up and pushes his penis into me. That way I get the full pleasure of orgasm with him inside me, and he usually climaxes just afterwards. It needs some pretty nippy timing, though!

SUPERTIP

If your partner is busy giving you some very enjoyable oral sex, but you are still conscious of that 'invisible barrier' stopping you from actually climaxing, try this. Using your own hand, manipulate yourself around the area of your pubic hair, almost as if you were masturbating. It's too high up to exert much pressure on the clitoris – and besides, he will be responsible for that – but once again the *illusion of control*, the illusion of being in your own familiar masturbatory position, is often sufficient to overcome that invisible barrier and bring you to orgasm.

I have found this tip quite invaluable.

PART THREE

CHAPTER FOURTEEN

TO FAKE OR NOT TO FAKE?

Counterfeit the sweet bliss with lying sounds . . . Only, when you pretend, see that you are not caught, win assurance by your movements and even by your eyes. Let your words and panting breath make clear your pleasure.

Ovid, *The Art of Love*

There is no doubt about it: for me, faking was a significant step in my success.

Do I hear cries of protest? Faking entails deceit and distrust and that sort of thing? I do hope so. There is nothing so encouraging as a big chorus of out-dated moral disapproval. For although faking remains one of the last real sexual taboos, thousands of women do it every day. The fact is that there are very good reasons for faking your orgasm, especially during your learning period. Faking can *help* you to achieve orgasm.

WHY DO WOMEN FAKE?

Let's face it, nobody *wants* to have to fake an orgasm. Why then do we do it?

There are many reasons. By far the most common is that we

fear to display our so-called 'inadequacy' in not being able to climax. We are afraid of being labelled *frigid*. There are many variations on this particular fear. Here is just a small sample of comments I have come across:

I always felt that because I couldn't come I wasn't a proper woman. I mean, imagine a man who couldn't ejaculate. I certainly wasn't going to advertise that, so I started faking.

I simply couldn't stand the snooty look when I told them I hadn't come. As if they were getting second-class goods. It's so much *simpler* to fake it.

I tried not to, because I always felt it was the wrong thing to do. My therapist impressed upon me that the idea was to build up a loving relationship, and that faking introduced deceit. So next week I didn't bother to fake, but Mark got really angry because he said I wasn't trying hard enough. I suppose that dumb psychiatrist must have really gone to my head, because then I confessed to Mark that I'd never had an orgasm. Wow! Did the shit fly! He said he felt that he was dating an iceberg, and left me a few days later. I changed my shrink.

You're caught: if you don't fake they think there's something wrong with you, and if you do fake some twit starts sounding off about it being the thin end of the wedge and underhanded. The only thing is to tell the twit to piss off, and keep faking.

I think I could have borne a man who got angry when he found out. I mean, then I'd have known he was a bastard and that would make things simpler. Even an indifferent man would be OK, in fact he would be best of all, because I could just get on with it myself. But it was Ben's endless little attentions that got on my wick. Always worrying about me and looking at me with pitiful eyes as if I had three arms or something.

For me it's very simple, when my husband keeps pumping away at me, in and out, my vagina gets sore. It's OK for the first ten minutes, but I just don't have that much lubrication. If I didn't fake I wouldn't be able to walk the next day!

Often when I had sex with my boyfriend, he'd compare me unfavourably with his previous girlfriend. If I wasn't writhing in ecstasies he used to tell me how hot she was. That upset me more than if he'd gone on about how beautiful she was. I felt really jealous. So I started faking so as not to be outdone.

Why do I fake? Oh, that's easy. I fake because I don't like doing it with my husband. Faking gets it over as quickly as possible.

What a dismal situation!

Another important reason why women fake their orgasms is the fear of upsetting their partner. Many men anxiously insist that the woman must have satisfaction – either because they are genuinely concerned, or in order to satisfy their vanity and prove they are a 'good lover'. It is one of the little ironies of our sexually liberated era of equality that men have come to demand that their partner have an orgasm *just as they do*. Or, in the words of Catherine Stimpson, an eminent feminist writer:

Men tried to invent a new, friendly, eager female sexuality in what has been called the sexual revolution of the sixties. But after that experimental decade, the feminist movement emerged to challenge men's motives, insisting that the command to be sexually warm was as oppressive as the earlier command to be cold and pure. The pressures that gave rise to those inventions remain.

This is part of the reason that women like Harriet fake – in order
to get a little peace:

> Sometimes I get really angry that he can have an orgasm
> and I can't. But if you are with a man who feels that he
> ought to give you a chance it can be very tiring. He might
> mean well – but to lie there while he keeps rubbing away
> at you, all the time expecting you to collapse into ecstasies,
> well it's hard work. It's also awkward – if he's been trying
> for ages and still you can't, there comes a point where it's
> very embarrassing to admit defeat and stop. I reckon it's
> simpler for everybody to fake it. He's satisfied, and you're
> as satisfied as you'll ever be.

Some women I've met even fake orgasms to be polite.

> If I've been for a nice evening out, to a smart restaurant,
> maybe to a show, I figure it's rude and ungrateful not to
> indicate you enjoy the sex that goes with it. Marilyn
> Monroe used to fake so as not to offend her partner, so
> why not me? You know what men's egos are like – and if
> you like the guy, why not? It costs you nothing.

I think if men knew just how *often* women fake they'd be
astonished. I can recall several occasions when men I've known
have let slip details of their partner's 'great' sexual responses –
when only the day before the woman in question has been
congratulating herself on her skill in faking.

I've also known of one or two men to shake their heads over a
woman faking, with sympathetic and understanding comments like
'She shouldn't feel she has to'. But when their partner doesn't
come, then, by God, don't these same men make a pained
atmosphere, if not get actively angry? It's a sad fact that when it
comes to sex, reality and ideals are a long way apart.

But faking orgasm in a relationship is not always intended as a
major deception. Sometimes it begins as a temporary measure, as
in Bella's case.

> When Larry and I first met I didn't want to disappoint him. I loved him a lot, he turned me on, and I was sure it was only a matter of days before I had an explosive orgasm. The trouble was, the days turned into weeks, then months. The orgasm never happened. How could I tell him I'd been pretending all along? I had to keep it up. Now I feel resentful.

In short, faking is a consequence not a cause of sexual difficulty. It is not so much a form of deceit, as one of defence. It does not exaggerate poor communication or sexual unease, it is only a response to them. In fact, with careful handling, it can, on the contrary, be the means to a far more open, honest and satisfying sexual atmosphere.

I have already explained how, in my own case, when I was younger it simply never occurred to me to fake orgasm. I was too naïve. I wish I had known, it would have saved me a lot of embarrassment, heartache and guilt. It was only when I set about devising this programme for myself that I realized faking could help me. I began faking orgasms quite deliberately. I decided it would be the first stage in my long haul – by buying me time to concentrate on myself.

And it worked.

HOW CAN FAKING HELP ME?

I have all along stressed the importance of a sense of *control* over your own body. By faking an orgasm you are taking the pressure off yourself, ridding yourself of anxiety. In such cases, contrary to what so many well-meaning people say, faking can *help* to stabilize a relationship. It requires a form of deceit, to be sure, and we would all prefer to do without it. But it is no use talking of ideals when the reality itself isn't in order. If having to announce your lack of orgasm makes you tense and worried, or causes friction between you and your partner, then it's often worth a little deceit to avoid what can be a major unpleasantness.

So do not frown on faking. It can be an invaluable aid to your progress, and it need not be any upset to a loving and caring relationship. In fact, it can do a lot to help breed stability and understanding. Once I knew that I didn't have to worry so much about the humiliation of admitting to my partner I was *not* going to climax, I was free to concentrate on my enjoyment during sex. Instead of constantly getting in a tizzy about the fact that in ten minutes' time my boyfriend would be over and done and probably starting to ask me difficult questions – and looking hurt when I gave him the truthful answer – I could relax. And relaxation, as you will have gathered by now, is an essential part of this programme. Furthermore, if the man feels you will *eventually* reach orgasm (i.e., your faked orgasm), he'll usually be prepared to go on a great deal longer than if he feels it's all for 'nothing'.

Naturally, I don't mean to say that you should fake whenever you feel the slightest desire to, or whenever you know you won't be able to have a genuine orgasm. I certainly don't think you should fake to be polite, or to pander to your man's vanity. If and when you fake, you fake *because it is helping you towards a more satisfying sex life*. On those occasions when you feel that the pressure on you to have an orgasm detracts from your pleasure and concentration, then faking may be the answer. These occasions are personal. I cannot dictate under what conditions your need becomes great enough: that is for you to decide. All I can do is say that you should not feel it is necessarily wrong or harmful to fake an orgasm. On the contrary, it may be the only way you can get that sense of ease which is so important to your progress.

Anna is assistant manager in a local insurance office:

> Faking did help me, there's no doubt about it. My husband is a really nice guy, but when we first met he didn't give much attention to my needs in bed – this was twenty years ago remember. We had a pretty average sex life I should think, though I never got aroused enough to have an orgasm. But we muddled along, and I was distracted by

my career. After we'd been married for several years, Harry picked up a sex manual. That got him thinking about what he'd rather taken for granted before – my satisfaction. He began asking me if I climaxed, and because I loved him I didn't want to lie. When I kept saying 'no' he felt he ought to put more effort into our lovemaking. That was OK, but it made me nervous, him always asking me, 'How was it for you, dear?' – I mean it's a bit of a joke question.

It got to really bother me in the end – but how could I say shut up when he was trying to be decent? I remember one evening I'd had a hell of a day out shopping and I came home and got into the bath tub. I took a drink in there with me, and I must have dozed off because when he came home I was still there in the bath. Watching him undressing while I lay there, I suddenly wanted him.

We got into bed, and I was thinking, yes, I bet I could do it this time I feel so good. Well Harry got on top of me and started away. We were doing really well and then he spoiled it all by saying, 'You really must have an orgasm tonight, darling, I'm determined to keep going till you do.' Privately I'd been thinking just the same – but as soon as he said it, I sort of froze. I knew immediately, with him watching for it, that I couldn't. At work they say that if you're presented with a deadline, your adrenaline rises and you really get going. Well, sure as eggs is eggs, that's not true of sex. I let him go on for a while, and then I thought, Oh bugger it, I'll fake it – and I did. He was thrilled to bits.

After that I faked it most times we fucked. I'd felt really angry that first time, for having to. But after a bit I realized that I'd bought time for myself. I'd get him to keep going for as long as possible which he was more happy to do now that he felt there was something tangible at the end of it. And now that he 'knew' I had no trouble climaxing, he left me alone more. Finally I could relax. And then I did do it: I climaxed. After that it got better

and better. I'm certain I would never have been able to
without that faking.

But there's more to it than that. Not only can faking put you at
ease, so that you may enjoy your sex as much as possible without
fretting constantly about whether you will or will not come at the
end of it, but by making good use of your ease you can *develop* and
train your sexuality so that you will learn how to have an orgasm.
For many, faking is the path to non-faking!

Some men are not concerned whether a woman has climaxed or
not, in which case this will not be your problem. If you know this
characterizes your partner, then it might be worth trying to get *out*
of the habit of faking (if you are already in it) or not getting into
the habit in the first place. Faking is only useful if you feel awkward
about admitting to not climaxing. There's no point in faking if you
feel perfectly at ease with him about your inability.

I certainly do not think you ought to fake an orgasm to help his
ego, or to be polite, but if faking an orgasm will allow you to be
yourself, then I believe it is justified. You will be free of the anxiety
of him asking constantly, 'Have you come yet?' You will be free to
concentrate on your own method of learning.

SURELY HE'LL KNOW IF I'M FAKING

That's what I used to think, but I was wrong.

The positive news (at least in terms of faking) is that most men
are lamentably ignorant about whether or not a woman has come.
In my experience those so-called Lotharios with vast experience
are often the worst. It tends to be men who have been in stable
long-term relationships who are the most sensitive and the most
acute.

But instead of taking my word for it, let men speak for
themselves:

This business of knowing when a girl comes is pretty vague and shadowy. It's open to a lot of misunderstanding, as well as out-and-out fraud. I would have to admit that I'm often not sure at all.

The subtlety of some women's orgasms can be deceiving. I usually try to tell by the partner's movements, a change of pace, quickening of breath, moaning, contractions, grip, affection, kisses, etc., but usually I am not sure.

I can never tell for sure ... I am always in doubt ... right now, since each woman seems to be different, it seems thoroughly baffling to me.

These are all from *The Hite Report on Male Sexuality*. Hite concludes that 'most men experienced a great deal of insecurity and confusion over knowing when – or whether – a woman had had an orgasm'.

HOW DO I FAKE AN ORGASM?

If you do decide that faking is justified, it is very important that you do it convincingly. Bear in mind that it *can* do damage to a relationship if he finds out and feels you've wantonly misled him.

If you haven't faked until now, it'll make him very suspicious to find you suddenly having orgasms to order. But think about it carefully: if you haven't faked until now, perhaps there's no need for you to start. Only if you feel it really would help you is it worth doing – *don't* start doing it just because you'd like to give him a little present now and then. It's you that needs the little presents, not him.

If, having thought about it, you decide that faking is indeed the lesser of two evils, then introduce it gradually. Naturally you'll have to be consistent. Fake it once, then leave it a few times. Then fake again, and so on.

Now you can't easily fool a sexologist in the laboratory with all his measuring equipment, but you can fool your partner any day. Remember, when you fake, the following points are important:

1. Your breathing – probably *the most* important indicator. Don't ring up one of those sex lines to find out how they do it, because they're grossly exaggerated. Any man who thinks that's your average orgasm sounds like he has unsavoury pastimes. You'll notice during masturbation that your breathing changes quite a bit during the lead-up to orgasm and during orgasm itself. Notice that it is not simply a heavy panting which erupts at orgasm and then vanishes. Almost as soon as you begin to masturbate it will change. Gradually it gets heavier and quickens quite a bit towards your climax, then takes a minute or two to die away. Avoid making it too rhythmic; vary the pace every now and then. During orgasms some women make a lot of noise, some go very quiet just beforehand, and then start gasping during it. And most women vary from day to day. There is no one way. All women are different.

Exercise 14.1 To be done *before* you begin faking. Get hold of a tape recorder. Switch it on to record, making sure the microphone is close to your face. Now lie down and begin a masturbation session. Then replay the tape and listen carefully to your breathing – you'll be surprised at how much it changes, without you being aware of it.

Exercise 14.2 Again tape record yourself masturbating. Then play it back and listen carefully. Now tape record yourself faking an orgasm. Can you tell the difference?

2. Vaginal contractions. Although some men say they can feel these, most admit they cannot. (Hite in fact specifically asked this question, and reported all negative replies.) This is good news for fakers. All the same, it's not a bad idea to rhythmically tense and untense your vagina a bit (you can do it three or four times at about one a second) at the moment of orgasm, just as you have noticed in your masturbation sessions.

Exercise 14.3 Masturbate yourself to orgasm. Just as you begin to climax, insert one or two fingers into your vagina. This will allow you to gauge the degree of the contractions.

Exercise 14.4 This exercise is nothing more than the Kegel exercises mentioned in Chapter 6 – that is, clenching and unclenching your vaginal muscles. It can be done at any time of the day or night, without anyone else being any the wiser. Like all muscles, the more you use those in your vagina the greater their tone will develop.

3. Erect nipples. Dr David Reuben really did the dirty on women when he wrote

> Erection of the nipples always follows orgasm in the female.
> In spite of heaving hips, lunging pelvis, passionate groans
> – no nipple erection, no orgasm. It is an accurate mammary
> lie detector – for those who insist on the truth.

We've had trouble with Dr Reuben's little sillinesses before. And, just as his nonsense about oral sex clammed me up for years when it came to cunnilingus, so this little gem was one of the reasons I never dared to fake – and so prolonged my misery in the face of men who resented my 'frigidity'.

There is, in fact, no need to be intimidated by this 'biological fact'. Like that age-old and very misleading test for virginity – the bloody sheet – erect nipples are *not* a reliable guide to orgasm. Believe me, I was so obsessed with Dr Reuben's announcement that I've studied it in detail.

I'll begin by quoting the most famous sexologists of them all, Masters and Johnson: 'There is no specific breast reaction to the experience of orgasm.' Those of you who are likely to show nipple erection at orgasm are also likely to show nipple erection when you are first sexually aroused.

If that's not good enough for you, the strength of the erection varies greatly not only from woman to woman, but from orgasm to orgasm. And if there are *some* days when nipple erection is minimal, then there's no reason why that shouldn't happen *every* day, is there? Also, remember that temperature plays a part in how nipples behave. On a cold day they will be erect regardless of orgasm. If you really want to impress him with the quality of your (faked) orgasm, have him make love to you in the snow, or on Brighton beach!

Also if the woman is lying on her back, gravity often ensures that any nipple erection is absorbed by the posture of the breasts, and can easily go undetected. Lastly, it is quite possible to engineer your position – or your clothing – so that he has no access to your nipples.

Exercise 14.5 Masturbate yourself to orgasm while standing up, in a *warm* room. This position will show you the *maximum* erection your nipples are likely to achieve through orgasm. (If the room is cold you won't be certain which is the orgasm and which the cold.)

Exercise 14.6 Now masturbate yourself to orgasm lying down in a warm room. Again see how your nipples respond. The chances are they will be far less noticeably erect than when you were standing up.

4. When faking, bear in mind also that the quality of any individual orgasm varies greatly. I've had orgasms (real ones, that is) that have had me panting and moaning in a most theatrical manner. And then the day after I've had others that, even though intensely felt, I have enjoyed quietly and passively. Be inventive. Vary it – fake some nights, but not others. Incidentally, in the list above I have not mentioned the so-called 'sex flush' that some women experience, simply because it is not a necessity of orgasm.

Some women have it *some of the time*, and others don't. So don't give it a thought.

Exercise 14.7 For the really brave: to hell with the Knitting Circle, get some close friends together and form an Orgasm Faking Circle. Try this one: each of you tape yourself masturbating alone. Now get together and play them back, so that you get a really good idea of just how much women vary. Once the initial embarrassment has worn off you'll have tremendous fun.

If your man has never heard you climax before, he will have nothing to compare it with. But remember, it is still worth taking trouble to fake accurately, because quite soon you really *will* be having real orgasms – and you don't want him to think that you're faking then! So remember:

THE GOLDEN RULE
In general it is always best to underplay it than overplay it.

If, when you do start climaxing, you find your responses are significantly more intense than those you've been faking, you can quite truthfully say to your partner something along the lines of 'It's got so much more pleasurable lately, darling.' Don't do too much of that heaving hips, lunging pelvis, passionate groans stuff. Use your ingenuity: tell him to stop once or twice, and wait, thereby suggesting that you have almost had your orgasm and want to delay it for a while. Later, when you've completed your training, you may find yourself doing this anyway.

Don't fake too soon in your lovemaking session or he'll ejaculate and you'll be left with nothing. Spin it out.

Remember: it is *not possible* to 'prove' that a woman has or hasn't had an orgasm (unless of course you're down there with a torch and some pretty fancy equipment).

And lastly, an invaluable piece of advice: time your faked climax to coincide with his own: he will be in no position to judge you!

QUESTIONS AND RESPONSES

Because faking is a controversial subject I've included here a selection of some common questions, together with my responses:

Q: *I've read your list of faking advice, but it's scared me. How can I possibly remember all that?*

R: A very good question, since the whole point of faking is to make you free from anxieties, not filled with new ones. That list covers all there is to know about faking orgasm. It's a connoisseur's list, if you like. All you really need to remember are the following very basic points:

1) your breathing;
2) don't overplay by heaving about, or underplay by lying dead still and then suddenly exploding.

Basically, as long as you are familiar with the chapter on masturbation you'll know what's typical of you. In general, the more emotionally involved you are with your partner, the more you'll want to get it right – a one-night-stander isn't really worth the extra effort.

Q: *What shall I do if he finds out I've been faking?*

R: It depends what you mean by 'finds out'. If he *suspects* you, but you have made up your mind that it is the right thing for you to do, then simply stick to your guns and insist you were not. He cannot prove it. On the other hand if the manner of his approach is sympathetic you may feel that now you would like to come clean.

If for some reason you feel he really has rumbled you (read your diary confessions, for example) the important thing to remember is *keep your cool*. Don't look guilty, or act guilty. Remember, nobody wants to have to fake. If you've been faking it's for a very good reason. And believe it or not, it's far more upsetting for *him* if you go all flustered and admit you've been 'dishonest'. Although in our initial hurt and anger we want to have the satisfaction of blaming someone, in the cold light of day it's easier to accept that there was a good reason for one's partner's 'deceit'.

So keep cool and talk quite matter-of-factly about it. Say, 'Yes, you're quite right I have been faking.' Explain the reasons. Tell him that he's touchy about his ego and that this puts unpleasant pressures on you. Tell him you can't do it, and that his hopes for you doing it only makes it worse. If he makes a great big issue out of being hurt and upset, it's high time you reminded him that it's *you* who need the sympathetic understanding, not him.

Q: *I love my husband, and I can't get over feeling guilty about faking. What can I do?*

R: Then don't fake. It's an *option*, it's not compulsory. That's why it's not part of the main programme. But if you do feel there are reasons for faking, then you must simply concentrate on the fact that by faking you are paving the way ultimately to greater success. Think of it as a temporary measure only, a means to an end.

Q: *You say that failing to have an orgasm is nothing to be ashamed of, yet you recommend faking. Surely that's inconsistent?*

R: I hope I have made it clear in the early chapters that being unable to climax is nothing to be ashamed of. If anybody is at 'fault' – and often nobody is to blame – it is our partners. In an ideal world faking wouldn't be necessary. I have introduced faking *because it can be a means to buy time and peace for yourself*. It is a temporary measure to help you along to total success, not simply a way of escaping the embarrassment of admitting 'failure'.

I cannot repeat this too often: *the only reason you should be faking is as part of a plan to help yourself.* If you are in any doubt about faking, ask yourself the question 'How is this helping *me*?'

CHAPTER FIFTEEN

FANTASY

PHEBE: Good shepard, tell this youth what 'tis to love.
SILVIUS: It is to be all made of fantasy . . .

(Shakespeare, *As You Like It*)

I am a great believer in sexual fantasy. It has helped me immeasurably in learning to achieve orgasm. It continues to help me. However good my sex life, fantasy adds that extra touch of colour.

Nobody should be ashamed of a bit of sexual inventiveness. In all cultures people who employ their imaginations are highly valued: storytellers, novelists, poets, filmmakers. Using our imagination in bed is just as wonderful, with even more direct results. Fantasy – particularly when carefully combined with reality – can be a crucial feature of satisfying sex. To quote one famous sex therapist, Helen Singer Kaplan: 'Sex is friction and fantasy.'

MEN ONLY?

Sexual fantasy is more commonly associated with men than with women. The reason is, to my mind, clear and dully familiar – long years of cultural restrictions upon female sexual behaviour have created deep-seated feelings of guilt or shame in thinking about sex. In a recent discussion three women admitted they would feel quite unsettled if they allowed themselves to indulge in a wild fantasy about being ravished by a sheik: it's the sort of behaviour that is still associated with unseemly and unnerving lust rather than respectable womanhood. (A fourth agreed that a sheik fantasy would unsettle her, but only because she normally goes for blue-eyed blonds.) Most men, however, because they are *expected* to behave in an aggressively sexual way, are quite happy to imagine *being* a forceful sheik ravishing a woman – even though when the climax is over they might feel a little guilty and even blush pleasantly (I always enjoy a blushing man).

In the early days of psychoanalysis, sexual fantasy was treated as a form of sexual deviation. Dreary old Freud saw it as undesirable escapism, a repressive blocking of the sexual instinct that could lead to psychosis or neurosis (and thus, presumably, back to being treated by Dr Freud). Even forty years ago it was assumed that for most women sex was the means to what they really enjoyed: romantic slush and motherhood. Their fantasies were supposed to be correspondingly limp. But today it is recognized that female sexual imaginings are as powerful and lusty as any male offering. Best of all there are scores of reports to show that sexual fantasy has a very positive effect both on individuals and on relationships. Recent studies have concluded that the frequency of sexual fantasy was an excellent indication of a person's sexual health and success with orgasm. Another researcher went so far as to conclude: 'sexual fantasies help many married women to achieve sexual arousal and/or orgasm during sexual intercourse'.

Interestingly (make of it what you will) it seems that in males, the younger they are the more they fantasize, whereas in females, fantasy is rare among young girls, but much more common among older women.

WHAT DO PEOPLE FANTASIZE ABOUT, AND WHY?

Some common female fantasies include sex with a man with a huge penis, with an innocent young boy, before an audience, with another woman, as a prostitute, with animals, with domination, with a friend or associate, with a group, or, just to make sure nobody's left out, with a stranger.

Genette is very forthright about her sexual fantasies:

I literally couldn't have an orgasm at all without fantasy. And I don't regret that. Fantasy's great. It lets you really make everything you can out of sex. While I'm being fucked I think of all sorts of filthy things. Sometimes I whisper them to Philip, and I can feel him begin to shake at the thought of the scene . . .

One of my favourites is that I'm a warden in a prisoner-of-war camp, Second World War. I walk into the room, and all the men are there looking unshaven, ragged, lean and grubby. Then there's me, all clean and sleek, and wearing a really tight dress with my breasts half showing. I walk down the lines, where the men are standing by their bunks. Somehow (I wonder why!) all the men that I actually notice are really nice looking – tall, noble. Being officers they are all very self-controlled, so the whole scene is very tense. I walk up and down looking furiously at them, a whip in my hand. I approach one man, my eyes bright with scorn and contempt. He, very anxious not to flinch, says nothing. I obviously inspect him, poking him here and there with my whip. Then my hand goes to his trousers. I unbutton his flies. Still he stands there. I order a box to be brought. Everyone thinks I'm going to indulge in some sort of torture. I order him to stand on the box. That means his flies are on a level with my face. I undo his trousers. I can feel him shaking. I take out his prick, which is in that lovely stage between limp and stiff – half hard, really big and flopping in a sort of arc – he's fighting to control it, see. I take it in my hands. I place it in my mouth, suck on it, harder and harder until the moment he ejaculates when I pull it out of my mouth and watch the semen squirt all over me. Still I show no emotion at all.

The majority of people fantasize in order to help themselves become more sexually aroused – an astonishingly high 46 per cent of females, and 38 per cent of males in one survey (Sue). Nearly a quarter of women said that they fantasized to increase their partner's attractiveness, whereas 10 per cent of the men and 15 per cent of the women weren't sure why they did it at all! The great beauty of fantasy is that you are creating situations that are liberatingly impersonal and conveniently imprecise. Perhaps most important of all, *you* have complete control.

Even so, of the many female fantasies I have listened to I was struck by how many involved the *woman* being in control of the situation with the man in varying degrees of helplessness. Erica's is another good example:

I'm a thief – that's right, a female cat burglar. The house I've got my eye on is a big Georgian pile, with landscaped grounds and naked statues. In the middle of the night I steal in through one of the upstairs windows. I'm in a black outfit, very tight-fitting with a black mask. I'm also carrying a large *screw*driver (well, what else?). I'm creeping quietly around filling my sack when I hear a noise. The person in the bed has woken up. By the light of a small bedside lamp I see it's a man. *Of course* he's good-looking – mid-thirties, slender, dark – and terrified.

Slowly and with the tip of the screwdriver I roll the bedclothes back. With one hand I reach for his pyjamas. As soon as he sees my hand he realizes I'm a woman. I undo the button. My fingers brush against his prick. For a long time I play with his prick, part teasing him, part threatening. Then I force him to lie back. I straddle him. I unzip my trousers in a special place, without taking them off. Pinning him down I move up and down on him, up and down, slowly slowly, then faster and faster. I satisfy myself totally. Maybe I allow him to orgasm – maybe I leave him gasping for relief – it depends how I feel. Now the dawn is coming up. I peel off his pyjama bottoms, drop them into my sack with the antiques, and slip out of the window.

Another noticeable feature of many such imagined situations is their *impersonal* nature: highly erotic, but no messing about with love and romance. Great stuff for fantasy – especially since nowadays the risk of AIDS makes such encounters in real life very risky. Erica Jong, in her wonderful novel *Fear of Flying*, describes one scenario of what she calls the 'zipless fuck', an ideal type of copulation in which passion itself and not the person of your lover is the issue. Her fantasy takes place in a second-class compartment on a 'grimy European train'. An attractive young widow in mourning is sitting there, along with four other rather unpleasant characters. At one of the stations a sixth person enters, a 'tall languid-looking soldier, unshaven, but with a beautiful mop of hair, a cleft chin, and somewhat devilish, lazy eyes . . . basically a gorgeous hunk of flesh.' He sits down flirtatiously next to the widow. After a while he slips his fingers under her thigh. She shows no reaction. The four unsavouries get off at a station. The man grows bolder, but still nothing is said. The train then enters a tunnel 'and in the semi-darkness the symbolism is consummated' and the young widow gets off at the next town.

> Zipless, you see, *not* because European men have button-flies rather than zipper-flies, and not because the partici-pants are so devastatingly attractive, but because the incident has all the swift compression of a dream and is seemingly free of all remorse and guilt; because there is no talk of her late husband or his fiancée; because there is no rationalising; because there is no talk at *all*. The zipless fuck is absolutely pure. It is free of ulterior motives . . . And it is rarer than the unicorn. And I have never had one.

Fantasies are rarely well focused. It is more a matter of skipping here and there, picking up bits of mood and sensation, repeating bits you like, avoiding those you don't, playing not only the role of yourself, but also to some extent the role of the other characters. Unless my fantasy is a daydream, and engulfs me entirely, then I don't ever have my whole mind on it – some portion of my concentration remains with the facts.

A huge number of women fantasize about people they normally know in non-sexual situations. I always look forward to hearing

Laura's latest, which invariably centres round her doctor. It's particularly entertaining because I know the doctor too, and I cannot quite envisage him in the sort of situations she does. I see him as a rather dry, greying middle-aged man; she sees him as a mysterious stranger, suppressing his sexual energies:

> I've got a midday appointment for something quite innocuous. Something wrong with my hand, say, and by some sort of not quite clear reason I have to take my top off and I can see him breathing more heavily but keeping up a deliciously professional air . . . In the end, of course, he breaks down and pins me against the wall. The interesting thing about it is that I'm half concentrating on the way he feels and half on the way I do. The real me is fantasizing about a sort of imaginary combination of the two characters.

SHOULD I FEEL GUILTY?

There is one aspect of fantasy that used to make me suffer agonies of guilt, and that was my constant desire to fantasize about being raped, or forcibly made love to.

While it worked wonders for my ability to have an orgasm, the rest of the day I felt dreadful. I was under no illusion that such a situation in reality would be anything other than terrifying and hateful. To indulge as amusement in a situation that has in reality ruined women's lives seemed outrageous. It came as a surprise and a relief to learn that some form of 'rape' situation is one of the commonest of all female fantasies. Writes Nancy Friday about women's fantasies in *Men In Love*:

> the single greatest theme that emerged was that of 'weak' women being sexually dominated, 'forced' by male strength to do this deliciously awful thing, made to perform that

marvellously forbidden act, guiltlessly 'raped' again and again.

As has been proven many times, the point of the fantasy is never to replicate the horror of real rape but to overcome inhibitions by imagining that sex is compulsory.

In my fantasy, of course, I could also exaggerate certain things I found pleasurable without having to feel worried that I was too demanding or perverted. That's why when I write about 'rape' fantasies I put the word in quotes. Unlike rape, the whole point of the fantasy is that you lead the situation in the direction you want it to go, but under the pretence of having it forced on you. You choose your partner, the location, the way he approaches you, etc. In short, in an imagined 'rape' *you* are in control, whereas a real rape is a situation of complete lack of control: the two are not only dissimilar, they are complete opposites. (It is interesting, by the way, that women tend to get appreciably more aroused from fantasizing than they do simply by watching an erotic film. I put this down, again, to the pleasure of being in control of the direction and details of the fantasy, even if not in control within the scenario.)

Recently a couple of researchers (Bond and Mosher) conducted a study specifically to help dispel the myth that women are secretly willing victims of rape. Using what they term 'guided imagery' – that is, tape recordings of specially constructed scenarios – they presented two types of scenarios to a group of female volunteers. The first was 'an erotic fantasy of "rape"', during which the women got aroused and reported 'interest, enjoyment and pleasure'. As the researchers conclude: in this imagined 'rape' 'the woman is *in control* because she enticed and permitted the man to "rape" her for her own erotic purposes' (my italics).

It was a very different situation with the second scenario – a realistic scene of rape. The women reported 'disgust, fear, anger, pain, shame and depression' – feelings very similar to those reported by rape victims themselves. So much so, in fact, that the article contained an ethical consideration of how to proceed in future with such tests.

In my own case I think my forced sex fantasies have as much to do with shame as guilt. Just as the idea of one's parents indulging in sex can be embarrassing and slightly distasteful, so I – and many women I've spoken to – feel something like that about themselves. One woman I know actually has nightmares about seeing herself in the mirror having sex, and wakes up hot with embarrassment 'as if I'd just walked down the high street on a Saturday afternoon completely naked'. So it's no surprise to learn that this woman's fantasies all centre around forced sex, which is liberatingly impersonal. Her marriage is perfectly happy, yet when she makes love with her husband she asks him never to use her name. It's a bizarre position for him, as he confided:

> Men who keep mistresses go through agonies in case they blurt out the wrong name in a moment of passion. I go through agonies in case I blurt out the *right* name!

Surveys have shown that nowadays very few women indeed feel guilty about the fact of fantasizing. What they do sometimes feel guilty about is indulging in fantasies involving sexual intercourse with someone other than their partner. While it is sometimes kinder not to make these known to him (unless by mutual agreement), it really is a waste of energy to feel guilty, because the very nature of fantasy means that your mind is in an ideal situation, able to mould events exactly how you want them. You are able to imagine the pleasurable involvement in a scene that in the messy, unco-ordinated real world would most probably be quite unpalatable. Fantasy is not infidelity, because the chances are a real-life encounter with the object of your fantasy would prove very different from your imaginings, as Dorothy's experience while working in an office in New York demonstrates:

> I used to work for a big firm of accountants. I was one of three personal secretaries that dealt with my boss. I think we all fancied him – he was tall, quite powerfully built with glossy dark hair just going grey at the sides. He managed to be distinguished and rakish at the same time.

After a few weeks working there I began to fantasize about making love with him: I usually imagined us on the boardroom floor, in full daylight, with my shorthand pad in one hand . . .

Then one day I had to stay late, because I was going out to the theatre afterwards, and I had an hour or so to kill. I got out my make-up and things and spread them about. I was sure everyone had gone home. I stripped off my shirt and was sitting on my desk in my skirt. Suddenly the door opened and – you've guessed it – he came in. I thought he'd get embarrassed and go away, but he didn't, he just stopped still and stared at me. Then he came over and without speaking he began kissing me. At first this was quite exciting. He took my hand and guided it inside his open flies. 'Take it, take it,' he kept saying. He'd shut his eyes and was sitting there blankly, while I was rubbing his dick for him. For just one moment I thought 'Creep'. But that thought quickly passed and we carried on.

Finally he rolled my skirt up round my waist and started playing with my pussy. He did it very badly, though he obviously thought he was cool. I was lying on the desk and he undid the top button of his trousers and they fell round his feet. He opened my legs and brought his dick up and pushed it inside me. At first I was torn between thinking 'My God, fantastic, I'm finally doing it with him' and a nagging sense of distaste. It wasn't the way I'd envisaged it. I had my legs over his shoulders and he was standing there, puffing away. What he didn't know was that reflected in the glass doorway I could see his back view – a bare arse, skinny legs and trousers round his ankles. He looked – well, a creep. No doubt about it this time. The whole thing was a bit squalid. I thought 'I don't even like this man, and here I am lying on a table with him jerking off inside me.'

What really made me mad was that when he came he took his dick out of me, and pumped his semen all over the blouse I was supposed to wear to the theatre. Well that's

**what comes of having fantasies – not much similarity! I
threw the blouse away.**

Another very striking example of the difference between reality
and fantasy is provided by Olivia. She's been with Adrian for
seven years, and admits that she is sexually very jealous over him:
'The thought of Adrian even looking at another woman gets my
teeth gnashing,' she admits. Yet Olivia has a regular, favourite
fantasy that she employs whenever she has sex with him. It helps
her to reach orgasm:

> **Quite simply it's Adrian with another woman. For some
> bizarre reason I find it incredibly sexy. All the while he's
> fucking me I transpose each little detail so that it's as if
> he's doing the same to her – only I'm watching through the
> keyhole. When I'm slow to climax I just replay the bit
> where he parts her legs, pulls her knickers down and
> enters her.**

Obviously there are odd occasions when, either through too
much to drink, bad lighting or because we trod on our spectacles
the day before, we find ourselves in bed with the *wrong man*, and
then fantasy provides very necessary escapism. Janie was invited
to a ball, where she was introduced to an impeccably mannered
European count, who kissed her hand and waltzed her round the
room. The lure of blue blood proved irresistible:

> **He took me back to his house in a taxi. I was so bowled
> over by the chandeliers, the Louis Quinze furniture, the
> Rockingham china, that I didn't notice him unbuttoning
> his corsets. A cigar-smelling, pot-bellied male sidled into
> bed with me. I had no option but to fantasize as hard as
> possible about *anything* that would take my mind off him.
> A just punishment for being a snob!**

On the whole, however, fantasies are valuable because they *enhance*
moods and sensations that are actually taking place.

Even during sex with your preferred man there are ways and ways of fantasizing. Lying back, forgetting about him and thinking through your favourite story like a daydream is a waste: a waste of your partner, a waste of a good fantasy, and a waste of companionship. For the purposes of orgasm, the best type of fantasy is what I have called 'blended fantasy'. I know it sounds more like a recipe than anything else, but perhaps in a way it is – a recipe for orgasm. This is when you successfully combine fantasy and reality. Instead of imagining a completely foreign scenario, concentrate on interweaving the reality and the imaginary, by making sure that every movement your partner makes fits in beautifully with what you're imagining. The ultimate sophistication of this 'blended' fantasy is for you and your partner to indulge in mutual fantasies in which you *both* play a part.

PORNOGRAPHY, EROTIC LITERATURE OR ROMANCE?

Close to the subject of fantasy is that of sexually stimulating literature. There has been for a long time a debate as to whether women are sexually aroused by romantic stories, or by the more explicit stuff. This 'more explicit stuff' can be divided into pornography and erotic literature. Andrea Dworkin (an American feminist whom I have only ever heard speak on television, and even then burst out in applause at the end of her lecture though there was no one but the cat to hear me) defines pornography in terms of sexually explicit material depicting violence against, or the subordination of, women. She believes – I think quite rightly – that it should be made illegal. Erotic material, on the other hand, can be just as hard core but it is without the enforced female sexual inequality and hence not so damaging to women nor so provoking to violence and domination for men.

Kinsey was one of these researchers who believed that women experience little or no sexual arousal when confronted with sexually explicit material, but require a romantic context. I've always been suspicious of this, partly because I've been turned on by explicitly erotic material, but also because the idea of women liking only 'romance' is yet another way of patronizing them, keeping them in an inferior position as the weaker, less physical, more gullible sex; in short, suspiciously in tune with the sexual sentiments of the 1950s, the decade in which Kinsey did his work.

I'm glad to say that Kinsey is now regarded as out of date – especially where his conclusions about women are concerned. In fact, on this level, there's some suspicion that he was a bit of a fudger of results although no one quite likes to say so. More recently a researcher named Jakobovits challenged Kinsey's results and found that, on the contrary, there was very little difference between men and women in this respect: they both got aroused by erotic literature. Later studies have tended to support Jakobovits' conclusion that the crucial element which affects the level of arousal is the explicitness of the sexual material rather than the presence or absence of romance.

Of course this romance/explicitness debate is difficult to prove either way. The big bar to conclusive results in women is – as I've said elsewhere – the fact that it is very difficult to monitor accurately female sexual arousal. We don't have erections to show unequivocally that we are feeling horny. The fact that female attitudes to sex scenes are changing – and coming towards a preference for more explicitness – is reflected in those stalwarts of women's romantic fiction, Mills and Boon. Nowadays the following type of scene is typical (and I should add that while this one is in itself sexually arousing, within the context of the plot it is very much more so):

He was already undressing her, his fingers deft on the buttons of her dress . . .

'Touch me, Beatrice.'

She wanted to resist, to tell him that she wasn't ready, but she was overwhelmed by the sudden rush of emotion sweeping over her as his hands swept back up over her body to ease down the fabric covering her breasts.

'You can't know how much I've ached to do this,' he told her softly, 'and this.'

He bent his head and she felt his lips gently caressing her breasts . . . He made a deep sound in his throat and moved his body deliberately against her, until the delicate friction made her cry out . . . His mouth left hers and she knew he was looking down into her unguarded face as he deliberately aroused her . . . His voice shook and so did his body, the fierce thrust of it within her own suddenly wildly out of control. She clung to him, hearing him moan her name, feeling the sudden quickening of her own flesh as it responded to his male need.

Tiny quivers of sensation built up inside her, a quivery shivery tension that wouldn't let her go, that drove her to incite him to take her with him to that place where the boundaries of flesh and mortality exploded in a vast shimmering ball of sensation.

(Frances Roding, *A Certain Spell*)

Obviously not a piece to please radical feminists, but it does make clear that the situation is changing with the times – that is, that the more economic, intellectual and sexual independence women achieve, the more likely they are to feel freely aroused by literature. Because the point here is not simply that the modern woman indulges in extra-marital sex, but that that sex is evocatively described rather than simply reported.

So if you need to 'get into the mood' before going to bed – or even before masturbating – then read a few pages of an erotic book. When I was still learning to have an orgasm I often used to give myself a head start by reading a sexy book while my partner was preparing for bed. In fact, those early partners were positively hurried into the bathtub. (I daresay they all now have hideous complexes about being smelly.) There is no doubt in my mind that erotic literature can be extremely helpful in this programme.

Exercise 15.1 This is really an exercise in timing and control. Find yourself an erotic book. Hold the book in one hand, and as you read masturbate yourself with your other hand. I want you to learn to *time* your climax with the most erotic moment of the book. This may seem a frivolous exercise, but it will stand you in good stead. Repeat it as often as possible – if you like, combine it with exercises in Chapter 7.

DIRTY BOOKS OR LITERATURE?

'Masturbate myself to orgasm with an erotic story!' you may be thinking. 'That's the sort of thing dirty old men in raincoats do.'

Well, perhaps they do it too. All I can say is, as an exercise and a way of sexual pleasure, it's a perfectly clean, useful, interesting and delightful thing to do. The books you read can be the sort of scruffy thing you pick up from the over-eighteen shelf, or they can be some of the more liberated works of great fiction that sober, white-haired academics daily analyse and comment on. They both have sex and sexiness in them aplenty if you know where to look for it.

In the bibliography I have included a list of possible books you might like to try. Most of them are ones you can get in perfectly respectable bookshops, and nobody will think you're anything but a broad-minded and serious reader when you buy them. When you get home you can skip all the non-erotic bits and get to the nitty-gritty or savour their genius slowly – whatever you like. I personally think that the context of the erotic bit is all-important, being fifty-five times more sexy if you've had to wait thirty pages for it. If you're not that patient, read the sober bits during the day and keep the hotter stuff for bedtime.

If you (like me) are also partial to the cruder stuff, then you can try the local sex shop. I used to go there quite often (some have a convenient back door for those who are a little shy), even though I had very mixed feelings about such places. Clearly a great deal of what they sell is highly degrading to women; but equally clearly some of what they sell I find highly erotic. The readily available videos tend to be just plain silly. I remember one in which two

girls seduced the milkman, amid much squealing and giggling: you could clearly see that they were only pretending to ravish him, and at one moment a flaccid little penis hove into view.

On the other hand I've also seen some highly explicit videos (mostly imported from abroad) which leave you in no doubt at all that sex is taking place. I'm always torn between the arousing sight of couples actually coupling, and disturbing thoughts about what the female participants are *really* feeling. Dawn found an excellent antidote: gay videos. She assures me that if you want to see some really good-looking guys, with positively *enormous* equipment (I can vouch for the fact that the heterosexual penises are almost always disappointing) try getting hold of one of these. Though the more explicit ones may not be quite your cup of tea, the milder ones often show attractive males masturbating. And there are no uncomfortable worries about what the women are having to endure.

Nowadays, I have to admit, my female loyalties keep me away from the sex shop; but then nowadays, when I am so much more practised at orgasm, I don't need that extra stimulation. Quite apart from ideological issues, the danger of sex shops is that you don't know who you'll meet there. My friend (who lives in a small town) never quite felt the same about her chiropodist after catching him gazing at a foot fetish magazine. She bravely continued to consult him because, as she pointed out, 'I ought to have guessed. I mean who else would *choose* to spend their lives with other people's feet? As long as he doesn't get *carried away* I think of it as rather flattering.'

Mail order is another option – you find advertisements in all kinds of newspapers and journals. That way you've only got to worry that the postman is reliable.

Literature can, of course, be erotic either explicitly or by implication. Jane Austen's *Pride and Prejudice* is not only one of the world's great classics but probably one of the most genteel novels ever written. Yet the sexual tension between the two main characters, Elizabeth Bennett and Mr Darcy, is dynamite. This strikes me as a book that hovers delicately between 'romantic' and 'erotic' – being far too forceful for the former, and a little too restrained for the latter. I don't believe there's a woman alive who having read *Pride and Prejudice* hasn't fantasized about meeting Mr Darcy in the woods. Rose's favourite is Thomas Hardy's *Far From the Madding Crowd*:

> I fantasize about being Bathsheba [the heroine] and having three totally dissimilar men in love with me. The dashing Sergeant Troy swishing his sword in the moonlight; the passionate, repressed Farmer Boldwood, and then that wildly sexy union with the shepherd Gabriel Oak at the end. It may not sound particularly erotic – and there's nothing sexually *explicit* – but when you've got so involved with the characters, you can't help sharing in their passions. I find it much more sexy than the cinema.

Another one of my favourite 'classics' is the eighteenth-century literary masterpiece, John Cleland's *Fanny Hill*. It is the story of an innocent young girl's adventures in a brothel, written in the most improbably novelettish fashion you can imagine.

> . . . his breeches, before loosen'd, now gave up their contents to view, and shew'd in front the enemy I had to engage with, stiffly bearing up the port of its head unhooded, and glowing red. Then I plainly saw what I had to trust to: it was one of those just true-siz'd instruments, of which the masters have a better command than the more unwieldly, inordinate siz'd ones are generally under. Straining me then close to his bosom, as he stood up fore-right against me and applying to the obvious niche its peculiar idol, he aimed at inserting it, which, as I forwardly favoured, he effected at once, by canting up my thighs over his naked hips, and made me receive every inch . . .

The whole thing is absolutely delightful, and if you like to fantasize about being penetrated by ridiculously large (and ridiculously colourful) penises, then this is the book for you.

THE CLASSICAL FANTASY

Just to show that there needn't be anything disreputable about reading smut and looking at dirty pictures, let me tell you about Annie's fantasies. She's a tall willowy woman in her thirties who works as a graphic artist designing book covers, advertisements and so forth. I recently visited her in her flat in Bristol where, over a bottle of Chianti, we got on to the subject of fantasy. 'Well, what's your favourite?' I asked her.

'Oh, that's easy,' she replied, and reached out to the bookcase and opened a large glossy edition of artworks. 'I think some of the most erotic stories in the world are the Greek classics,' she explained, flipping over the pages and showing me illustration after glorious illustration, many by the great Renaissance masters. 'Most of my fantasies come from the Greek myths,' she continued. 'Marvellous stories, handsome gods – look at that torso – it's fantasy in all senses of the word: sexual as well as escapist. I must admit I do tend to envisage the gods themselves as any man I'm particularly interested in at that time. What I particularly like is that however lewd you make the fantasy, it never seems squalid. Also, you can read them on the train . . .'

So, next time you want a helping hand when your man makes love to you, buy a book of the Greek myths and ponder Zeus's unusual seduction techniques.

After all, you can embellish with your own special details . . .

CHAPTER SIXTEEN

KNOW
YOUR ORGASM

Whoever said orgasm wasn't important for a woman was undoubtedly a man.

(woman quoted in *The Hite Report on Female Sexuality*)

In this chapter I'm going to go into the nature of orgasm in more depth. I must have looked up the word itself in over a thousand books. Enormous volumes professing to investigate sexual behaviour often don't list it, rather as if the authors had barely heard of the subject, and suspect it might belong to another discipline – politics, perhaps, or some new particle found by the high energy physicists.

Other books list it, but only one or two very brief entries. You can just see the writer fiddling with the word: 'Orgasm? Again? Oh dear.' And then, after a cup of coffee and a few worried paces about the room, he returns to his desk and crosses out the reference altogether. 'Most likely it was a mistake.'

Recently the situation has got a little better. Sex research has become respectable and scientific; huge, confidential studies of the average person's sexuality have become popular – and since the average person in private is significantly more informative than the specialist in public, our understanding of the female orgasm has vastly increased. Feminism, aside from enforcing greater scientific objectivity, has helped to make sex *interesting*, and not just the subject of giggles and derision. Another advance is that animal behaviourists no longer focus entirely on the male sex of the species.

But although the complexity of the female orgasm has finally begun to excite widespread professional interest, our understanding of it is still slight. The female orgasm remains one of the most beguiling sexual mysteries of our time.

WHAT EXACTLY HAPPENS DURING SEX?

Many of us know what orgasm feels like, but you'd be surprised at just how much is going on inside our bodies. The sexual response cycle of the female (like the male) is commonly divided into four phases: excitement, plateau, orgasm and resolution. (Other classifications are possible, but this one, due to Masters and Johnson, is the most widely accepted.) I'll describe each phase briefly, partly because the way a given person responds during any one of these varies widely – there is no 'correct' or 'incorrect' way – and partly because the medical terminology is enough to make one feel quite queasy.

In the *excitement* phase, heart rate, blood pressure and respiration all increase, and the muscles also become more tense. In certain parts of the body – those typically associated with sexual excitement – there is an increase of blood supply which may make those areas redden and grow warmer. It is this that is responsible for increase in breast size, nipple erection and the so-called sex flush that occurs in some women.

The genitals undergo major changes during this phase, although the vast majority of people do not notice most of them. The clitoris, vagina and labia minora all increase in size due to more blood supply. The vagina also responds by producing lubrication which allows easier penetration of the penis, and helps sperm survival by neutralizing the vagina's natural acidity.

The *plateau* phase is really a misnomer. It is not that everything levels off until orgasm, but that most of the responses begun in the excitement phase continue to change, though at a slower rate. Meanwhile, the clitoris is retracted under the clitoral hood. The phase does not last long – a few seconds, to several minutes at most – although an extended period can be very pleasurable and often followed by a relatively intense orgasm.

During the *orgasm* phase heart rate, blood pressure and respiration all reach their peak, and are accompanied by involuntary contractions of the outer third of the vagina, and often also of the uterus, rectal sphincter and urethral sphincter. There are usually between three and fifteen contractions, occurring about every four-fifths of a second to begin with and then slowing down.

The most annoying aspect of orgasm itself is, of course, that it's over so quickly – a matter of seconds rather than minutes. Roberta gives an excellent description:

> Just before I come there's this slight pause as if I'm on the edge, just about to teeter over but not quite making it. It's almost like the drawing in of breath before a sneeze – such a quiet thing to happen before so loud a noise. I know what I'm in for and I'm desperate for it to happen, and I know I can't stop it and that I have just a brief second to wait . . . and then I'm falling. It starts in my groin, a touch of pure, agonizing pleasure which suddenly pours forth and grips me for an instant, and then submerges me in a sea of release. I'm mixing my metaphors, but a decent orgasm makes it impossible to do anything else. It can be such an intense feeling. Before orgasm I was moaning and moving around because I wanted more sex, more this, more that. But during orgasm I'm on my own; I'm groaning because of all that I'm letting go – all the sexual tension that I wanted to build up so much beforehand, all the tension in the world . . . Occasionally it's a feeble affair. Still nice, of course, and not to be sniffed at, but without the explosion.

During orgasm, many women stiffen, become rigid and don't look at all as if they're enjoying themselves. There's an excellent murder mystery, *Rough Cider* by Peter Lovesey, which I thoroughly recommend, in which an important twist of the plot hinges on just this oddity. Other women make all sorts of evocative noises while they climax, as the following delightful episode from the life of the sixteenth-century adventurer Sir Walter Raleigh shows:

> He loved a wench well; and one time getting up one of the mayds of honor against a tree in a wood ('twas his first lady) who seemed at first boarding to be something fearful of her Honour, and modest, she cryed Sweet Sir Walter, what do you me ask? Will you undoe me? Nay, Sir Walter! Sir Walter! At last, as the danger and the pleasure at the same time grew higher she cried in the extacey Swisser Swatter! Swisser Swatter! (John Aubrey, *Brief Lives*)

After orgasm (or orgasms), there is a slow, reverse-order return to normal which is termed the *resolution* phase. The enlarged vagina and labia minora diminish, the clitoris reappears, lubrication ceases, heart and breathing rate decrease, and blood pressure lowers. There's usually a feeling of relaxation, calm and emotional closeness.

Description by women of female orgasm are very rare in literature, because erotica over the centuries has been written almost entirely by men. The following piece comes from Mary McCarthy's *The Group*:

> She struggled against the excitement his tickling thumb was producing in her own external part; but as she felt him watching her, her eyes closed and her thighs spread open. He disengaged her hand and she fell back on the bed, gasping. His thumb continued its play and she let herself yield to what it was doing, her whole attention concentrated on a tense pinpoint of sensation, which suddenly discharged itself in a nervous, fluttering spasm; her body arched and heaved, and then lay still.

The intensity and sensation varies not only between one woman and the next, but between one orgasm and another. And, as I have already said, although many people go mad in their descriptions of orgasm, it can just as easily be a pleasant but nothing-to-get-het-up-about experience. In fact it's one of my main complaints that sex manuals tend to glorify orgasm to a positively intimidating degree. As one married woman confided, 'I get so worried that, much as I enjoy my climaxes, they never seem to be so deeply *significant* as some writers suggest.'

Of course a good orgasm is a profoundly satisfying experience, both physically and emotionally – especially if you're fond of your partner. But there are also scores of occasions for thousands of women when the earth doesn't move, it's quickly over and all we want to do is get dressed and have breakfast. It's only by acknowledging the mundane side of orgasm that we can really appreciate the peaks.

DO ANIMALS HAVE ORGASMS?

Now this *is* a fascinating subject.

To some extent the problem of why women have orgasms (and why they have difficulty with them) is connected with the problem of the female orgasm in other species. If animals have them, that implies it's a much earlier evolutionary addition to female sexuality than if they don't. But it was only in the 1970s that non-human females began to attract much research. Before then it was wrongly assumed that males were the interesting sex, while females simply hung around passively waiting to have babies.

In looking at animals, the first question is what constitutes an orgasm? In males, at least, you'd think that was an easy matter. But no, because ejaculation and orgasm are not necessarily one and the same. It may be quite possible (who knows?) for a male monkey, dog, hyena, kangaroo or whatever to ejaculate without experiencing any of the psychological sensations commonly associated with orgasm in human males.

How much harder, then, to decide about the female. After all, the bespectacled scientist can't *ask* a copulating female gorilla if she's having an orgasm. The researcher who works outside the laboratory can only sit quietly in the bush with his binoculars and packet of sandwiches watching and listening for sexual behaviour to see if anything strikes him as familiar. The scientist in the laboratory is a little better equipped. He must attach wires to the female in appropriate places. Once she gets going with a male he must register changes in blood pressure, heart and breathing rate, in muscular tension and hormone levels. Now he must analyse them to see if they fit in with human behaviour during orgasm. If most of the changes fit the human pattern, then the evidence for orgasm is pretty compelling.

For non-primates, the evidence is inconclusive. Female mammals have a clitoris, which may be stimulated during copulation, but by any account female orgasm is rare, either because in many species orgasm simply isn't possible for the female, or (as the very existence of a clitoris strongly suggests) because the circumstances are rarely right. The interesting thing – especially for our purposes – is that most researchers seem to assume that orgasm is *a potential that all female mammals have.*

For non-human primates the situation is happier. Because gradually, apes and monkeys all over the world are being ruthlessly exposed in their moment of sexual ecstasy. In 1971, female rhesus monkeys were brought to orgasm *not* by their own mates, who (in common with too many of the male animal kingdom, alas!) suffered dreadful premature ejaculation, but by the researcher himself boldly stimulating them (I hope they thanked him). In 1979 a researcher reported actually witnessing an orgasm in a female gorilla – and, while we're on the subject of gorillas, back in the 1920s there was a romantic case of cross-species attraction. A female gorilla named Congo used to grasp men's hands and use them to masturbate herself. On one occasion the famous animal psychologist Robert Yerkes narrowly escaped being raped by Congo.

In 1980 four Dutch scientists recorded uterine contractions, changes in heart rate and facial expression comparable to those in humans during orgasm in some female stump-tailed macaque monkeys – although the notable fact that immediately springs to my mind is that macaques are blissfully free from inhibitions (*four* Dutch scientists). But, in order to get stimulation to last sufficiently long (the male macaques also suffering premature ejaculation) the Dutchmen had to arrange an encounter *between two females*. Five years later their finding was supported by studies of macaque monkeys in the wild. Just watch the pages of your favourite sex journal to find out who will be next.

Masturbation occurs frequently in non-human female animals, as most pet owners are aware. Cats and dogs on heat often rub their vulvas against objects – sometimes objects which you'd prefer they left alone. I remember being ravished by an eager female Alsatian when, aged about thirteen, I wandered into the local tobacconist to buy some sweets. 'Well, we *are* wearing our mini skirts today!' exclaimed the shopkeeper, as if that somehow explained it. Since such behaviour (the dog's, I mean) serves partly for stimulation, and partly to leave a distinctive scent mark to attract males, it was rather fortunate I didn't meet a male Alsatian on the way home.

But my favourite example has to be captive female porcupines, who sometimes hold a stick in one forepaw, straddle it like a broomstick, and then walk around the cage dragging it along the ground so that the bumps and vibrations can gently excite them.

WHY HAS THE FEMALE ORGASM EVOLVED?

It's easy, of course, to explain why the male orgasm has evolved. In bald evolutionary terms, it is to the advantage of the species (at least during times when there is not overpopulation) to encourage the male to deposit semen frequently, and thus ensure reproduction. The very simplicity of this idea makes woman's capacity for orgasm difficult to explain. After all, according to the scenario, it's only necessary for the woman not to refuse, or be unable to refuse, intercourse. Physical weakness and/or a certain degree of enjoyment are all that's needed. Climax, says the pondering evolutionist, seems to be taking things a little too far.

Some researchers consider that the female orgasm helps to increase 'pair-bonding' between husband and wife. Sexual gratification is supposed to make emotional attachment between partners stronger, and by encouraging a stable, happy family unit the young have a better chance of survival. It's no surprise that this theory is held by researchers from widely different professional backgrounds – after all, it is the least adventurous and most socially respectable one that fits the bill. Hite does not support it.

Mary Jane Sherfey's theory is much more exciting, although (predictably) less widely held. In *The Nature and Evolution of Female Sexuality* she argues that orgasm – multiple orgasm even – was once the norm for women; so much so that men considered it needed suppressing:

> Primitive woman's sexual drive was too strong, too susceptible to the fluctuating extremes of an impelling, aggressive eroticism to withstand the disciplined requirements of a settled life . . .

Because, biologically speaking, women are able to have unlimited numbers of orgasms one after the other, our distant ancestors were able to go from partner to partner enjoying themselves without limit – and where does that leave society? Far from encouraging pair-bonding, Sherfey conjectures that the female orgasm was ruthlessly suppressed because of its disruptive influence. Sexual repression of women therefore became a key characteristic of the development of civilization, and women's ability to have orgasms has suffered accordingly.

There is indeed historical evidence to show that in societies the world over women's sex drives have been considerably suppressed. Stone Age art indicates that 20,000 years ago there was no clear differentiation between the social power of women and men. Furthermore, cave paintings concentrate much more on the woman's sexual organs than on the man's, suggesting that the woman's sexual role was particularly appreciated.

But changes have taken place since then. About 10,000 years ago humans began to understand that sexual intercourse – and not simply lying in the moonlight, or appeasing the gods – was necessary for pregnancy. This of course raised the status of the penis; and our not very enlightened ancestors began to consider the woman as merely another type of fertile soil into which he planted his all-important seed.

Other theories state that female orgasm has a reproductive purpose, helping to draw the sperm up towards the egg, while some researchers claim it has the opposite effect and actually blocks the sperm! And then of course there are those who believe it serves no particular function at all, but is very pleasant all the same.

Take your pick.

MALE VERSUS FEMALE ORGASM

Is there a difference between orgasm as experienced by men and orgasm as experienced by women? Hard to judge, of course, unless you've tried both, and sex-change patients are hardly typical examples. The authors of the *Arabian Nights* assumed the female's pleasure to be the greater, but the best one can say for certain is that verbal reports of orgasm by both men and women are very similar indeed.

However, while most men report that one orgasm is pretty much like another, women tend to experience a great range of feeling, from the highly intense to the comparatively mild. In my view this all adds to the interest of women, but then I'm biased. Another difference is that while men generally find their first orgasm the most intense and any subsequent ones less so, with women it is the other way round. While on the subject I cannot resist quoting this perfectly leaden description of male orgasm from Ernest Hemingway's *For Whom the Bell Tolls*:

For him it was a dark passage which led to nowhere, then to nowhere, then again to nowhere, once again to nowhere,

> always and for ever to nowhere, heavy on the elbows in the
> earth to nowhere . . .

Aren't you glad you're a woman?

The interesting thing is that as we in the West become more
sexually liberated (probably more so than ever before in history)
and less tolerant of the traditional inequalities between the sexes,
the difference between male and female desire and ability for
orgasm is rapidly *decreasing*. Studies reveal that there is practically
no difference between young men's and young women's desire for
intercourse. If this surprises you, bear in mind that other factors
can mask these essential similarities. For example, women are
slower to warm up for sex (and, as some partners may have failed
to notice, slower to cool down). And, because of their potential for
pregnancy, women have far more at stake each time they have sex.
It is very much in their own interests to select their partner with
care.

In fact many researchers are quite convinced that women have
stronger – though more readily suppressed – sex drives than men.
Masturbation is commonly considered the best indication of sexual
potential, and as we have seen women can easily masturbate to
orgasm as quickly as men. Many can also have multiple orgasms,
which is something very few males are capable of.

THE CLITORAL SYSTEM AND THE PENIS

We are accustomed to thinking of the male genitalia as very
different from that of the female. I have made the point at various
times in the book that this obvious difference contributes to many
of our attitudes. Dr Sherfey, however, points out that although the
genitalia of the two sexes may seem very different, there are in fact
remarkable similarities.

She describes the clitoris as merely the small visible part of a
hidden *clitoral system*. The penis can be compared to this system,

both in terms of size and response to sexual stimulation. As she so nicely puts it:

> **We may say that the external genitalia of the female are homologous to the entire penis split open along its under-surface and the split-open scrotal sac.**

And during sexual excitement (in Hite's words) 'the only real difference between men's and women's erections is that men's are on the outside of their bodies, while women's are on the inside.'

Both have analogous regions – the *crura* and the *corpora cavernosa* – which become filled with blood during sexual excitation and serve, in the case of the clitoral system, to contribute to the enlargement of the vagina, and in the case of the penis, to erection. Also, just as there are sets of muscles to help with the erection of the penis during the excitement phase, so there are homologous sets of muscles which retract the clitoris during the plateau phase. The rhythmic contractions of the vagina during orgasm are caused by muscles which have precise counterparts in the man, causing contractions that force the ejaculation of semen – what's more the contractions are at the same rate, i.e. every 0.8 seconds.

In terms of size, the penis and the clitoral system are about the same when excited. The clitoris itself, far from being the focus of sexual responsiveness as so many assume it to be, is just the tip of the iceberg (to use a most inappropriate metaphor).

THE VAGINAL AND CLITORAL ORGASM

The notion that women experience more than one type of orgasm began with Freud. His idea was that women who have not yet accepted their passive sexual role or learned to come to terms with penis envy, experience clitoral orgasm. He associated this type of (supposedly not very satisfying) orgasm with masturbation, which he considered to be stimulation of the female penis counterpart, i.e. the clitoris. Mature women, on the other hand, experience a vaginal orgasm due to vaginal stimulation during intercourse. Unlike clitoral orgasm this is supposed to be more satisfying because it occurs with women who have adapted comfortably to their sexually inferior status and receptive role!

It is an obnoxious theory, although for its time not unusually so. And to be fair to Freud, though its reasoning is absurd, the idea is motivated by more than simple male chauvinism, which explains why the vaginal–clitoral myth continues to bumble along despite having been disproved and discredited.

Part of the trouble was that during Freud's time there was no material available on the sexual responses of the average woman – all studies, by the likes of Krafft-Ebbing, Havelock Ellis and Freud himself, being confined to cases of sexual oddity and perversity. It was only in 1953 that Alfred Kinsey – a soft-spoken, kindly academic who had a fondness for bow ties, and whose previous professional experience of females was confined to gall wasps – finally published the first sex survey of the average woman. Because it revealed so much – bad and unconventional – about American sex lives, and because it raised sex to a scientific status, his results were viciously attacked by certain political elements; Kinsey died a broken man three years later. Small wonder that it wasn't until the mid-sixties that Masters and Johnson conclusively showed that the two types of orgasm are one and the same: sexual intercourse stimulates the clitoris indirectly by putting moving pressure on the clitoral hood.

Ignorance has done more than anything else to keep the vaginal–clitoral myth alive. Woman's sexual organs are complicated and difficult to understand. The remarkable discrepancy between the ease with which women can have orgasms during masturbation, and the difficulty so many seem to have during intercourse – although now known to be a result of either insufficient clitoral stimulation, or the need to learn sexual skills – might well lead less critical scientists to suggest the existence of two types of orgasm. Even today it is promoted from time to time because general acceptance of sexual equality is still very young and tender, and among some members of the psychoanalytic world there continues a goodly amount of male chauvinist priggery.

But the hard fact is this: although most orgasms for women are *induced* by clitoral stimulation, they are always *expressed* by the vaginal muscles. The orgasms may vary in intensity and sensation according to whether there is intercourse or not, but this in general is a result of the different circumstances rather than a different type of orgasm.

Hite talks about a further type, the 'emotional orgasm'. This she defines – of necessity, rather loosely – as 'a feeling of love and communication with another human being that reaches a peak, a great welling up of intensity of feeling' that may have sundry physical manifestations. I'm with her wholeheartedly when she advises that, as long as women are not pressured into using these as a substitute for real orgasms, they are just one more means of enjoyment.

IS THERE AN EQUIVALENT OF MALE DIFFICULTY WITH ORGASM?

Yes, there is. (I'm not talking about impotence and failure to get an erection, which of course is very common, but simply failure to ejaculate.) But it's so rare that even those few researchers wanting to pursue it have had difficulty in finding individuals to study. One report (Mann) cites 'religious orthodoxy, male fear of pregnancy, negative feelings toward or lack of interest in the partner and, in a few cases, evidence of homosexual orientation or maternal dominance'. For those men who had once been able to ejaculate normally, and had lost the ability, a stressful event could usually be traced to explain the problem: one failed after his wife was unfaithful, another after his wife's mother and sister moved into the house.

This same researcher noted another unusual factor: namely that several of these men masturbated in an odd manner that had very little similarity to coitus. But then if (as in one case) you're accustomed to getting your pleasure by striking the shaft of your penis forcefully with the heel of your hand, I suppose it's hardly surprising that a woman's body doesn't provide quite what you've been used to.

Occasionally men also fake orgasms, usually when they're simply afraid that they won't be able to ejaculate. And in this department, apparently, women are as easily misled as men.

THE G-SPOT

Having said all this, there is, famously, recent (inconclusive) evidence for a further type of orgasm resulting from stimulation of the so-called Grafenberg spot by deep penile thrusts during intercourse. This is not the vaginal orgasm of Freud, but some researchers believe it to differ from the clitoral orgasm.

The G-spot is a lump on the wall of the vagina about an inch or two inside the opening, toward the stomach. According to the theory, it is the female counterpart of the prostate. At first, stimulation of it causes a desire to urinate, but this is quickly replaced by sexual arousal and enlargement of the spot, which may lead to orgasm. In some women the orgasm is accompanied by the ejaculation of a fluid chemically very similar to semen.

But the theory has undergone a scientific battering since it was first publicized in the early 1980s. There are a number of alternative explanations for both female ejaculation, and for the fact that certain areas in the vagina feel better than others. And these are perfectly in accord with not having a G-spot at all.

Perhaps the most interesting aspect of G-spot discussions is that they give a good idea of the topsy-turvy, indecisive nature of academic sex literature. Different sorts of orgasm are all very interesting to read about, but it's much better to forget them when you get into bed. At the moment they are little more than the suggestions of scientists at play.

FEMALE EJACULATION

There is a great deal of debate still about so-called female ejaculation. Some say it doesn't exist, others argue over what exactly it is. From personal experience I am convinced that it exists: a small amount of fluid given off at the moment of orgasm. Some men believe they can feel it being ejected, high up inside their partner.

I am equally convinced that it's not, as some researchers persist in arguing, urine, but something much more akin to the normal healthy vaginal lubrication. It's not only colourless and quite inoffensive, but many men find it extremely arousing. One other thing: it has been observed to occur mostly in women with strong pubococcygeus muscles. So, if you're really interested in it, turn to page 70 and start exercising! Then you can pursue your own research on the subject.

NOCTURNAL ORGASMS

We're all familiar with male nocturnal emissions, or 'wet dreams' as little boys call them. Did you know that women, too, sometimes have orgasms while they are asleep? Just how often this happens is hard to gauge. Men know they have had a nocturnal orgasm even if they don't wake up during it, when they find the bed is wet. Because women leave no such tell-tale signs, female nocturnal orgasms seem comparatively rare. If, however, women are able to experience them without waking up, they could be quite common. As it is, most of the research has, by necessity, been on those instances when the woman awakes during the orgasm. A *Playboy* survey reported that approximately 40 per cent of women admitted having had at least one – a figure less than half that of males.

What is especially common is for women to wake (often after a highly sexy dream) feeling maddeningly on the *point* of orgasm, only to find that they badly need to pee. I've lost count of how many times that's happened to me – usually just at the tantalizing moment in my dream when I have succeeded in bedding whoever it is who has inspired the dream. It's enough to try the patience of a saint.

I'd always assumed that nocturnal orgasms would be more prevalent among women with a repressive attitude to sex: if you don't allow yourself sex in the normal way it has to come out somehow, sort of thing. I was surprised to read that in fact nocturnal orgasms are in general associated with women who hold liberal and positive attitudes towards sex. They are, however, predictably more common amongst those who have been without sex for a long while – in prison, divorced, etc. Interestingly, male nocturnal orgasms are most common during the late teens and early twenties, whereas women peak during their forties.

DO APHRODISIACS HELP WITH ORGASM?

Aphrodisiacs – potions that increase sexual desire and ability – are a lot of fun. Nothing else gives quite such a sense of how delightful, ingenious and silly people can be about sex. But, sadly, they're rarely all they're cracked up to be. However, for the woman on this programme it's useful to know something about the subject, and also about possible *an*aphrodisiacs – those substances which might make orgasm more difficult.

It's no surprise to learn that most aphrodisiac experiments – both ancient and modern – have been centred on men and male sexuality. Very much less work has been done on substances with respect to female sexuality, and less still on women's ability to reach orgasm. After all, those men who were interested in female sexuality were usually keen just on getting the woman to want it more in the first place, rather than concerned with her satisfaction.

Among all the commonly used drugs and medicines there is

little evidence that they either increase or decrease women's ability to climax. Alcohol is surely the most familiar 'aphrodisiac', although from the point of view of orgasm it is a mixed blessing. As Shakespeare puts it:

> MACDUFF: What three things does drink especially provoke?
> PORTER: Marry, sir, nose-painting, sleep and urine. Lechery, sir, it provokes and unprovokes; it provokes the desire, but it takes away the performance.

On the plus side alcohol reduces inhibitions and 'sex guilt'; it's also useful in slowing men down. But drink too much and the bloke is out of action altogether. And, in similar fashion, for women its desensitizing effects can make a difficult orgasm impossible. When I was first beginning my training I found that I became quite skilled in judging how much I wanted to drink. Spirits put the kibosh on the whole proceedings, but one to two glasses of wine helped me to overcome inhibitions without interfering with my responsiveness. If I drank much more it meant no climax. Nowadays I find I can go to a party, get pretty merry and still reach orgasm, albeit more slowly.

Nicotine is best classed as an anaphrodisiac: not just because smokers pong, but because there is clinical evidence that smoking may be associated with impotence in some males, probably because nicotine reduces blood flow and thereby makes erection more difficult. As to the effects of smoking on female sexuality, there is – guess what? – virtually no information whatsoever. Why not try your own research? If you're thinking of giving up smoking, make a chart (similar to that in Chapter 5) of your own sexual responses both before and after stopping. It won't be precise enough to satisfy a scientist, but that doesn't mean it can't be valuable to you. And if you plan to send your questionnaire responses in to me, why not add your nicotine findings as well? Bear in mind, however, that unpleasant symptoms associated with first giving up the habit will probably, in themselves, have an adverse effect on your desire for sex.

Oral contraceptives deserve a mention here. Despite the fact that the pill is thought by many people to have encouraged sexual promiscuity by removing fear of pregnancy, it does put some women off sex. Its progesterone content can cause reduced clitoral sensitivity, and may outweigh the effects of oestrogen which can help to increase libido for women with low sex drives. 'It's certainly an effective contraceptive,' moaned one man. 'It's put her right off doing it at all.' If you suspect the pill may be reducing your sex drive, try a different type before you give up altogether.

So-called 'street drugs' such as cannabis, LSD, cocaine have long been reputed to have a variety of dramatic effects on sexuality, and by implication, orgasm, but despite these extravagant claims the hard evidence in favour of their aphrodisiac qualities is pretty limited. In most cases harmful side-effects will immediately, or eventually, outweigh any positive aspects. There is no question about it: the opium, heroin, morphine group of drugs severely depresses sexual desire and responsiveness.

That leaves the more fanciful aphrodisiacs. Despite current medical scepticism, almost every culture in the world has, or has had, a lively aphrodisiac tradition, with every kind of concoction from haggis to crocodile teeth. Some, such as bull's testicles, are used because of their obvious association with sexuality, and I'm sure human testicles have been used at some time, although it's best not to think about that. In North Africa, the Siwanese men sometimes conceal some of their own semen in their partner's food. I once shared a flat with an oriental woman who whenever she had a new boyfriend began consuming large quantities of vanilla. When I asked the reason, she explained that vanilla pods resembled the female genitals, so that according to the doctrine of signatures – the ancient belief that resemblance indicates similar powers – they would certainly increase her sexual arousal.

If your partner's lovemaking isn't all it might be, the *Kama Sutra* advises that he drink boiled clarified butter every morning during spring. If this doesn't work he can try boiling a goat's testicle in sugared milk. And if, poor fellow, he still finds himself unable to satisfy you he must resort to piercing his penis with a sharp instrument, increasing the size of the hole by inserting small pieces of cane and fruit stalks, and then washing the swollen member all over with liquorice and honey.

Spanish Fly is one of the classic aphrodisiacs, supposedly effective in vastly increasing female libido. In fact Spanish Fly is the poison cantharidin, and one thousandth of an ounce is a fatal dose. No wonder the Shakespearian euphemism for orgasm was 'dying'. The reason it's become so famous as an aphrodisiac is that the cantharides irritate the genito-urinary tract – in short it makes your vagina itch like mad so you need something up it to soothe the annoyance. A chemist called Arthur Ford accidentally killed the two women assistants whom he'd intended to seduce, and nearly did away with himself when he shared some coconut ice with them into which he'd pushed a huge amount of Spanish Fly. with a pair of scissors. The autopsy revealed that the victims' internal organs had been literally 'burned away'. Nowadays, cantharides are used mainly to remove warts.

Until recent centuries the mythical mandrake was extremely popular as a sexual stimulant, notwithstanding the fact that it doesn't exist. It grows only at the foot of a gibbet, glows in the dark and gives a lethal squeal when you pull it up. In order to avoid death on collection, a dog should be tied to the plant, and then called once the collector has retired to a safe distance. There are several real plants known as mandrake, and these are mentioned in the Song of Solomon as a cure for sterility, and in *Genesis* as the bribe with which Leah induces Jacob to sleep with her.

Ginseng is particularly popular in the East, and nowadays rather a fad in the West. Since the shape of the root can vaguely resemble the human form, according (once again) to the doctrine of signatures ginseng should be beneficial to the whole body. And, indeed, if you pop into the local outré health food shop, you'll find it recommended for just about everything. Analysis of the biochemical components of ginseng root has shown that it contains stimulants which are remarkably effective and low in toxicity, unlike coffee or tea. On the negative side, a recent survey suggested that it can cause diarrhoea and skin eruptions – and you can't get more unromantic than that.

I'm sorry to be such a wet blanket, but the fact is it's easier to find anaphrodisiacs than their happier counterpart, and if anybody tries to sell you an orgasmic concoction, denounce them to the office of fair trading. Exercise and practice will work infinitely better and at a fraction of the cost. That's not to say, however, that your own imagination can't do service as the best aphrodisiac in the world. A year or two back, feeling my sex life had become distinctly drab, I consulted an ancient book of herbal remedies and devised my own love potion to end all love potions: plants picked by moonlight, stirred about with dew, and a few magic incantations muttered over them before I gobbled the lot. *Of course* I felt sexier that evening – wouldn't you?

CHAPTER SEVENTEEN

CONDITIONS THAT CAN AFFECT YOUR ABILITY TO REACH ORGASM

We have seen how difficulty with orgasm can be overcome by training. However, there are some conditions – medical and otherwise – that can severely, or totally, impede your enjoyment of sex and reaching orgasm.

I have deliberately kept this chapter brief: its purpose is simply to alert you to possibilities. For a fuller discussion of medical conditions and how to treat them I strongly recommend Denise Winn's very helpful book *Below The Belt*. Some others, more broad-ranging, are suggested in the bibliography.

VAGINAL INFECTIONS

As every woman knows, there is a whole host of conditions – some rare, some distressingly common – that affect female genital regions: thrush, gardnerella, herpes, trichomonas, chlamydia, gonorrhoea, etc. Pain in the vagina, itching, discharge or an unfamiliar smell are the most obvious symptoms, although not present in every case. If you have any one of these go to the doctor: most are treatable.

Thrush merits a special mention because it is one of the most common conditions preventing women from fully enjoying sex. It is a fungus which may already exist in your vagina without causing trouble. However, a change in the vaginal acid balance can cause it to run rampant and result in an infection: you'll know because instead of the normal vaginal secretions there will be a lumpy 'cottage cheese' type discharge, a bad smell and sex will be sore. Indeed many women know thrush is on the way simply because of a recognizable discomfort during sex. Thrush can be caused by many things – the pill, the IUD, even sex itself; it frequently appears after a course of antibiotics.

At the first sign of symptoms stop having sex and get treatment: it is fairly easily cured by three days of vaginal suppositories (now available without prescription), although it has a maddening tendency to return. Because it can crop up so unexpectedly I make sure I always have one or two extra courses of medication handy, although strictly speaking you should always get a doctor's examination in case it's something else.

CYSTITIS

Cystitis is an infection of the bladder, and one of the most miserable commonplace conditions women can get. It causes a burning pain in the bladder and a nasty feeling of constantly needing to pee. Sometimes there is fever as well, or an uncomfortable feeling in the groin. Most women suffer from cystitis at some time in their life, some are repeatedly plagued with it. The trouble is that familiarity has made many women blasé. For many years I had attacks: horrid while they lasted, but as soon as the antibiotics began I was OK. Of course, the antibiotics also brought with them thrush, but that was a blessing in comparison with cystitis. So I went along, not especially careful to take steps to prevent it. Until one day after an attack I took my usual course of antibiotics – and it *still* wouldn't go away. Suddenly a comparatively minor complaint became something quite frightening that I could not shake off.

Angela Kilmartin's excellent books – now almost classics on the subject – helped me a lot and, eventually, I overcame it. I don't mean to alarm you – just to say that this condition can be so horrible, and so damaging to a sexual relationship, that it's well worth taking deliberate precautions against ever getting it in the first place.

Always keep your genital area clean – and make sure your hands are clean when you touch yourself there. Wear cotton, not nylon underwear. Use only fragrance-free soaps, deodorants or talcs in your genital region, as all these can cause allergies. Perhaps the most important piece of advice is when you go to the toilet *always* wipe from front to back – never the other way around. Bacteria that are perfectly harmless in the gut cause havoc in the bladder. Believe me, such precautions will stand your sex life in good stead.

OTHER CONDITIONS

In general sex should not be painful – if it is there's probably something wrong. I've already mentioned the various infections. Very vigorous sex can make you sore inside, and you may have noticed that this often happens at the start of a new relationship, when you're so keen on each other you do it three or four times a day. Also, for women who have not had sex before, an unstretched hymen may be the cause. Being tense can also cause difficulties, by causing us not to relax the vaginal muscles properly.

Lack of sufficient lubrication speaks for itself. It can come about through tension, because your partner is using a condom, by your lack of oestrogen, or simply because you're made that way: despite what the sex books say, not all aroused women get sufficiently wet. If it worries you, consult a doctor, but in most cases it's simplest just to use saliva or lubricating jelly such as KY.

Vaginismus causes strong, involuntary tightening of the vaginal

muscles which can make penetration extremely painful or impossible. Its origins are psychological, but not to be sniffed at because
of that – the result is as physical as a pile of bricks. It might be
because you have certain fears about sex, or because you feel angry
towards your partner for some reason, or because you feel guilty
about something. One woman suffered vaginismus because she
knew her mother disapproved of her boyfriend, and was cured only
when she became strong enough to break free of the mother's
overpowering influence. Helen Singer Kaplan's *The New Sex Therapy: Active Treatment of Sexual Dysfunctions* discusses the subject at
length and suggests a physical treatment which you can learn. You
will probably also find that by working your way through the early
steps of this programme which do not involve penetration, the
condition is greatly improved.

Pain deep in the pelvis might be due simply to your partner's penis
being too large (see below), or for various treatable medical reasons
about which you should consult your doctor.

There are also non-painful, physical reasons that may hold back
your progress with orgasm:

Slack vaginal muscles (as often results from childbirth) can limit
your sensitivity for two reasons: one, by reducing the friction
between the penis and the vagina, and two, because slack muscles
mean a less vigorous blood flow. By exercising the vaginal muscles
and keeping them strong and fit, you greatly increase the flow of
blood, while at the same time probably improving both the ease
and the intensity of your orgasm. These Kegel exercises are
discussed in Chapter 5.

Intercourse during pregnancy is almost always harmless, but there
are a few unusual circumstances in which penetration and/or
orgasm can cause problems, particularly if you've had miscarriages
before. Talk to your doctor if you feel worried, because your sexual
reservations may well be unjustified and interrupt your progress to
orgasm for no good reason.

The Missionary Position (woman lying on her back, man on
top) can be difficult or uncomfortable in late pregnancy. Although

this is helped by putting pillows under your back, it's probably more advisable to use other positions.

FACTORS AFFECTING YOUR PARTNER WHICH AFFECT YOU

Premature ejaculation is discussed in more detail in Chapter 10. This troublesome condition can be treated by well-established and successful methods. I recommend Helen Singer Kaplan's book *The New Sex Therapy*.

A large penis may sometimes be *too* large. By hitting the cervix it causes pain deep down, particularly in certain positions: man entering the woman from behind, or woman lying on her back with her legs drawn up. Indeed, in some positions, even an ordinary size penis can be uncomfortable – if your coil is badly fitted, or if you have constipation, for example. Putting a pillow between the two of you can help. Also make sure you are fully aroused before penetration, because arousal causes the cervix to move back.

The French (of course) devised a special protection against an outsize penis – something called a *bourrelet*, which was 'a small silken pad, stuffed with cotton and rounded in shape, with a hole in the middle corresponding in size with the circumference of the penis for which it was intended'. So if this is your problem, perhaps you could make your own . . .

CHAPTER EIGHTEEN

A CHAPTER FOR MEN

There is no such thing as an uninvolved partner in a marriage where sexual dysfunction exists.

(Masters and Johnson, *Human Sexual Inadequacy*)

The Hite Report on Male Sexuality reveals that men's greatest complaint against women is that they don't want sex often enough:

Too many women find sex disagreeable, painful, messy, even disgusting and resort to pretexts to avoid it.

I would like to have a wife that was *interested* in sex, more often, more variety, more times.

I could be supremely happy with her if she were excited about me.

I would change sex primarily by increasing my wife's urge, or by decreasing my own. That's the biggest problem.

More. I just want *more*.

If this is true in your case, there is one overwhelmingly simple remedy: *make sex for your partner more enjoyable*.

Now imagine the following scene. It is evening. You and she have been to the theatre, then out for a meal. You have sat opposite each other for two hours, watching each other, anticipating the moment when you will make love together. You go home; you undress, turn out the light. You begin to make love. Just as you are getting really worked up, your partner climaxes, pulls away from you, rolls over happily and goes to sleep. When you show distress, she actually has the gall to suggest that it's your fault!

That is what sex is like for many many women.

The circumstances may be very different, but the fact remains that thousands upon thousands of women do not get as much out of sex as their partners do. Which, considering the vast female *potential* for orgasm, is tragic. For both sexes.

The Hite Report on Female Sexuality reveals the astonishing fact that approximately 70 per cent of sexually active women have trouble with orgasm. Either they have *never* climaxed, or they can do so only now and again, or with effort.

It is sometimes difficult for men to realize just what sexual frustration means for a woman. The fact that a sexually aroused man who has not climaxed has a large and very prominent erection staring his partner in the face leaves her in no doubt of his state. But sexually aroused women have nothing obvious to *remind* men that they may be feeling terrible inside – frustrated, angry, disappointed.

The fact that for a variety of reasons most women don't like to be insistent about their sexual needs only compounds the situation.

It is not true that women as a category have lower sex drives than men; or that women don't want orgasms as much as men; or that women are less sensual than men. Believe me, women can have sexual needs just as powerful as men's, even if they are shy about insisting on them. One bad experience can leave a woman feeling that sex is not all it's cracked up to be. Quite often years of putting her partner first, sexually, leaves a woman believing that she doesn't have much of a sex drive herself – or, the self-deprecating comment I've heard so often, 'not one that really matters'. The fact that these women have not had the *opportunity* to enjoy a satisfying sex life is quite a different matter. Seeing your partner satisfied night after night, when you are left to look after yourself, creates not only sexual tension but emotional discord: after all, it is supposed to be a *partnership*.

Most generalizations about the sexes are crude and unhelpful. But it *is* true to say that, sexually, women tend to defer to men, to give their partner's sexual needs more importance than their own. (For a more detailed discussion of this, turn to Chapter 4 'Women Take Control'.) There are many reasons for this, but at the heart of them all are centuries of conditioning.

Whereas, on the whole, men are able unselfconsciously to make the most of sex for themselves, it is very hard for them to realize that women often find it difficult to do so. I've lost count of how many times I've heard a male friend say to me, 'She only has to ask. But she doesn't seem to mind if I go right ahead and enjoy myself.' If you add women's reticence about being assertive in the bedroom to the fact that, physiologically speaking, women need more careful and patient sexual attention, it's not surprising so many individuals are dissatisfied with their partner's lovemaking. Of course I am not suggesting that this is necessarily so with you. But I do know the problem is much more widespread than our 'liberated' era would suggest.

A large part of this inability to appreciate a woman's sexual needs and frustrations is due to the fact that the male and the female orgasms are not simply two versions of the same thing. They evolved at different times, and they involve different factors. Unlike the male orgasm, the female orgasm is extremely subtle and sensitive. In the right circumstances, with a partner who understands and satisfies her needs, a woman can realize a huge sexual potential that under less favourable conditions might never have got the chance to show itself. In fact, scientists and sex researchers have found that, if anything, women have *higher* sex drives than men. Biologically speaking women can climax again and again, even while the man lies exhausted on the bed. Their second and third orgasms are usually more intense than their first. The reason they don't enjoy sex as often as men is because sex hasn't been *made* as enjoyable for them. I should, however, add that I am speaking of women as a category. Individual women vary in their sexual needs just as much as individual men.

IT'S NOT SIMPLY HER CONCERN, IT'S YOURS TOO

It is certainly not my intention to cast unnecessary doubts on your own relationship. After all, 30 per cent of women are apparently quite satisfied with their sex life. I want to suggest some means whereby, if you are concerned that your partner is not getting as much satisfaction as you are, or even that you would like to be able to give her *more* orgasms than she is already having, you can help. Your relationship will benefit, not only in the bedroom, but in all sorts of non-sexual ways as well.

Women's difficulty with orgasm is not simply due to men's inadequate understanding of their needs. It sometimes happens that everything is absolutely as it should be, and the lover is doing a wonderful job, yet still no orgasm. Perhaps she is feeling tense about contraception; perhaps a hundred different things. But inadequate understanding is certainly a very important factor, and if men really knew how to make love to a woman, women's difficulty with orgasm would be vastly diminished. This says nothing about men being less sexually adept than women, it is simply a consequence of the fact that women's sexuality and orgasms are more complicated. Not better, or worse – different. Just as women need to *learn* how to make the most of their sexuality, men need to *learn* how to become successful lovers. In certain cultures this is recognized. Men and women are *taught* how to make sex satisfactory for both partners; and in those cultures *all the women have orgasms all the time*.

It takes some courage for a man to pick up a book like this. Yet this chapter is relevant to *all* men, whatever the status of your current partner in regard to orgasm. If she is having trouble with orgasms then it is obviously important for you. If you would like to make love with her more often, then understanding the subtlety of her needs is the clue to achieving it.

I think if men knew just how rare and desirable a considerate and attentive lover is they would fall over themselves to learn how to be one.

WHAT CAN I DO TO HELP?

Ideally you should read the rest of the book. Chapters 2, 3 and 4 are the most important. These will explain in greater detail that while men's orgasms are comparatively straightforward affairs, women's are complex. 'A bloody nuisance' we call them when we're feeling pissed off; 'delicate and exquisite' when things go well. As you're reading the steps of the plan, attempt to understand why they progress as they do, and what they say about a woman's needs. Don't feel shy about this. Men and women psychologists and researchers alike still regard female sexuality and the female orgasm with awe: they are baffling subjects.

You will also learn that for all the sex on TV, in the films, magazines and on the bookshelves, there is still a great deal of ignorance. Age-old sex myths still persist. Almost everyone I've ever come across, male and female, believes in a number of complete sexual falsehoods that sex researchers have been trying to dispel for decades. Did you know, for example, that many men still fear masturbation – not, as in the olden days, because they worry they will go mad or blind, but an updated version of that superstition that they will fall ill through losing too much protein and body fluids? Did you know that most women don't find a large penis any more satisfying than a small one? Did you know that the clitoris should hardly ever be directly stimulated? Do you have any idea how many women feel forced to fake their orgasms out of desperation and guilt?

This ignorance is nothing to be ashamed of – communication between men and women about their intimate needs and feelings is notoriously difficult, and our society is still one that tends to giggle about sex rather than discuss it – but it is something to be corrected as soon as possible.

If you're interested in finding out more, try *The Hite Report on Female Sexuality*, a survey of the sexual attitudes of 3500 American women of all ages and backgrounds. It's a very good way to put yourself in the picture over women's attitudes to sex.

ASKING YOUR PARTNER

Books can tell you only so much. As I have tried to make clear in this one, the one thing that *is* certain about women's sexual behaviour is its diversity. Ultimately, the only way of finding out your lover's individual needs is to ask her. I cannot overstress how important this is.

'I can't ask,' protested one man when I gave him this advice. 'She'd think me such a wimp. I mean, men are supposed to *know* about these things.'

This seems to me one of the tragic misunderstandings between the sexes. Believe me, it is men and not women who cling to this idea of being 'macho' above everything else. No woman worth her salt will be put off by a man because he takes the trouble to ask her what she likes, rather than painfully plunging ahead.

Think of it the other way round. I remember when I first tried to give a bloke manual sex – absolute disaster! I'd seen pictures of penises in the books (pored over them, in fact) and they looked simple enough. But I'd never considered the difficulties of lubrication and pressure until the time when I was suddenly faced with one in the flesh, and I was too embarrassed to ask what I should do with it. So I simply took a deep breath, clasped the presented object tightly, and began rubbing away hell-for-leather until his agonized cries stopped me. At a teenage party my schoolfriend Anne bravely plunged her hand down the trousers of a man she was canoodling with in a dark corner – only to be hideously embarrassed when her rings got caught in his pubic hair!

If asking outright really is beyond you, do as recommended in Chapter 12 and 'ask' with your hands. That is, explore her gently, tentatively, and listen and watch her response. Just because a sex manual suggests something does *not* mean your partner will automatically enjoy it. Some women, for example, love having their nipples sucked, others hate it.

Techniques for enjoyment may take time to perfect. But remember that there is nothing more off-putting to a woman than a man who assumes he knows exactly what she wants – puts his own 'technique' into effect – and succeeds only in making himself foolish. And there is nothing more *enjoyable* than a man who takes care to find out what she, personally, wants, and how best to give it to her.

TELLING YOUR PARTNER

If you have a permanent partner who has (or whom you suspect to have) difficulty with orgasm, be cautious about mentioning your involvement in any 'help' programme.

One of the biggest mistakes sex therapists, counsellors and sex manuals make is assuming that just because a couple are a couple that they need to 'tackle it together'. Certainly you are both *involved*. You may well want to tackle it together. But that is not the same as saying that you should necessarily work at it in unison. Of course there are couples that will prefer to do this, and to follow this plan together. But I particularly devised the plan for women who wanted to be completely independent.

There is a very good reason for this: by announcing your participation you may make her feel that the pressure on her to have an orgasm has increased; and it is precisely this sort of pressure that can make it hard for her to have an orgasm in the first place.

If your partner does want to enlist your help, then that should be her prerogative. Don't feel resentful if she doesn't. This has nothing to do with lack of love or failure of sympathy between you. Sometimes the opposite in fact – the very closeness of the relationship can, paradoxically, make one feel shy. Far better to make it easier for her by quietly training yourself to become as satisfactory a lover as possible, and letting her get on with her training programme in her own way.

THE ESSENTIAL QUALITIES OF A GOOD LOVER

Before you start spluttering about my incredible nerve in trying to teach you your job, stop and – once again – think of it the other way round. Would you object to a woman having done a little reading first, to try to find out the best way to please you in bed? And remember, most women would have much less difficulty with orgasm if their lovers knew their business. Read about those marvellous Mangaian boys in Chapter 2 and you'll see what I mean. That's not to say that all you have to do is learn a few skills, read up some oriental texts on how to delay ejaculation and – Bingo! – problem over. Eavesdrop on any gathering of women who have got on to the subject of sex and you'll soon realize that there are all sorts of qualities that most of us prize in a lover. Of course there are exceptions, but the following suggestions I think most women would agree are a good starting point.

1. *Understand what sexual influences – superficial or profound – are at work*: her worries about contraception, fears about not looking attractive enough, guilt about wanting sex desperately but being unable to find it satisfying.

You may not like the feel of rubber and decide to forego the condom just this once when you make love, but you could be spoiling *her* chance of orgasm, because she will be worrying about getting pregnant. *You* may prefer to have the light on during sex, which results in *her* not being able to relax because she feels 'too fat', or her breasts are 'too small'. The fact that *you* don't think she has these faults is not always enough to set her mind at rest. Black stockings and suspenders may look sexy, but they can be bloody uncomfortable to wear. When you make love, think carefully about this sort of thing – give her the opportunity to feel *really* relaxed.

2. *Encourage equality*: the second biggest complaint among Hite's men was that women didn't take the initiative. This is the result of another great misunderstanding between the sexes, because many women resent having to play submissive, yet feel they need to

because that's a woman's role and to do otherwise would seem 'cheap' or 'unfeminine'. Recent studies have shown that women find erotic stories in which women take the initiative significantly more arousing than those in which men do. And part of the reason why there seems to be some connection between education and ability to orgasm is because better educated women tend to be more assertive about their sexual requirements. Having an element of control in the lovemaking does wonders for a woman's enjoyment. *Allow and encourage* your partner to take the initiative. Many women want to but don't dare because they are afraid of putting men off, or of being labelled 'crude', 'pushy', 'forward'. Indicate that you enjoy it when she takes control or initiates sex.

3. *Learn to control your own orgasm*: what is premature ejaculation? Quite likely you thought of it as a medical condition with which some unfortunate men are afflicted, which makes them ejaculate immediately they enter a woman – sometimes even before. The definition given by Masters and Johnson, in their pioneering work on sexual difficulties, might surprise you:

> [The authors consider] a man a premature ejaculator if he cannot control his ejaculatory process for a sufficient length of time during intravaginal containment to satisfy his partner in at least 50 per cent of their coital connections.

In short, 'premature ejaculation' refers not just to the speed with which a man climaxes, but also to the satisfaction he affords his partner. A mature lover is able to continue intercourse long enough so that *both* partners have a chance to be contented.

Of course, Masters and Johnson's definition is a little too simple. Some men suffer badly from what we traditionally think of as the medical condition of premature ejaculation – to the extent of climaxing within a few seconds, *despite* their best efforts during intercourse to prevent it. With proper training and sympathy it can be corrected.

But for many men the ability to last long enough to give

maximum pleasure is either a skill which they could acquire with a bit of effort, or a capacity which they don't bother to use, preferring instead to climax as soon as they feel the urge; premature ejaculation is then no longer a medical condition, it is simply idle and selfish.

The simplest and most common way to delay ejaculation is to spend more time in foreplay arousing and relaxing your partner. In fact this is so much the usual way that it has led to the common misconception that women in general *prefer* extended foreplay as opposed to extended intercourse. But this is untrue – the fact is that extended foreplay is for many women the easiest way to get the proper amount of attention.

It is much better if you can develop techniques to delay your ejaculation *during* intercourse. There are several ways of going about this. First you can slow everything down. Women tend to approach their climax more gradually than men: the speed of your movements matters less than their constancy, rhythm and duration. Twenty thrusts at a sprint will usually have less effect than ten minutes of slow build up. If you find yourself growing too heated, then stop or withdraw: men cool off far quicker than women, and when you begin intercourse again your partner will have kept much more of her original level of arousal than you have. Anyway, in the meantime you might try gently using your hand or mouth.

Robert developed a useful method that helped both him and Miriam:

> Instead of moving your penis in and out, you can keep it almost stationary inside the vagina and gently move your hips. This way you continue to excite your partner's clitoral region by the motion, without exciting yourself at the same rate.

One trick to delay ejaculation recommended by the orientals of old (who devoted a lot of time to sexual skills) is this: if you feel yourself to be on the point of ejaculation, relax all the muscles in your body, particularly your buttocks. The novelist Henry Miller recommended filling your head with mechanical thoughts (try multiplication tables) to prevent orgasm, while one ancient Chinese philosopher found an infallible method was to imagine himself balancing precariously on the branch of a tree!

There are various books (see the bibliography) which have been written to help men overcome the problem of premature ejaculation. And lastly, a useful tip if you are planning to make love later in the evening and worry you will come too quickly: masturbate an hour or two beforehand.

4. *Never rush your partner*: if a woman finds it difficult to have an orgasm, then it doesn't make it any easier if the man is coaxing her on like a racehorse. Greta explains:

> Do you know what the single biggest bar to orgasm is for me? Worrying that I'm taking too long. Normally I have no trouble climaxing, I just need a bit of time. But if I start to worry that I'm taking too long then I'm caught, because if I worry then it takes me longer which makes me worry more, etc. Often the whole thing is ruined and I have to give up in frustration. Then I get really angry.

In regard to women who are slow, or have difficulty with orgasm, it is very difficult for a man to strike a balance between going on long enough to allow her to climax, and knowing when she'd prefer to give up. After all, going on too long can be painful and dispiriting. All you can do is be as sensitive as possible to her mood in general.

5. *Never think that all sex must end in orgasm*: this is a very common mistake. Women in particular are sensitive to the fact that sex is *not* simply about orgasm – each minute of it should be a pleasure in itself. Chapter 8 deals with this in more detail.

A really good lover should encourage sexual situations with his partner which *don't* end in orgasm for either of you. Caress and fondle all you like, have intercourse, even; but let it be recognized by both of you that neither intends to have an orgasm. If you can set up these situations and make them a regular, familiar occurrence, this will probably do more to help your partner than anything else.

The idea is to draw attention away from the subject of orgasm, to make it something about which you can both feel relaxed, not to insist on it being the focus of your activity. If you announce that you're going to make her come, or make a great show of waiting for her 'to do her bit', then you'll simply make both of you feel unpleasant, and consequently it'll be much much harder for her. Only bad lovers think satisfactory sex is simply a matter of sufficient thrusting and climax; a good lover makes his partner relax and enjoy each moment as it comes rather than making her fret over whether or not she'll have an orgasm.

6. *Experiment gently with manual and oral techniques*: both manual and oral sex are a great deal harder for men to do to women, than for women to do to men. A woman's sexual area is no simple matter: as a *female* friend of mine says earlier on in the book. 'I'm damned glad I don't have to make love to another woman. I wouldn't have the first clue about how to arouse her, or where to fiddle!' Chapters 12 and 13 will make clear that it's not simply a matter of finding the clitoris and rubbing away merrily. The clitoris is a much more sensitive organ than the penis, and too much concentration on it can be extremely painful. You must learn to excite it indirectly, by rubbing or massaging the region around it, and over it when it is not exposed. Once again, no two women are alike, and you should be aware that what one woman may find pleasant another might not like at all. But if you do learn the skill of giving good manual and oral sex, you will be a great prize.

So, if you don't quite know how to give your lover manual sex, oral sex, anything – *ask*. Even the most sexually sophisticated man will have to ask (either directly or by knowing how to read the signs his lover is giving him) what a woman wants. Asking will not only make you more accomplished and her more satisfied, it will also help to build up a supportive atmosphere that will greatly help her if she has difficulty, and improve the quality of your sex life in general.

7. *Don't be demanding*: it is a standard female complaint that men who demand sex, or expect it as their due, are both off-putting and offensive.

If you want to make your partner feel her best and think of you as a really enticing prospect, don't be pushy. Don't go shoving her hand into your trousers – I can tell you from personal experience that that's a real turn off! And if you want oral sex, *don't* demand it, or start pushing her head down into the right region – there's a world of difference between demanding or strongly hinting for a blow job and making it clear you love it when she offers. Sexual demands are threatening and they build up resentment, particularly if your partner has difficulty with satisfying her own sexual needs. As Robina puts it:

> I love performing oral sex on my boyfriend. Give me half a chance and I'm down sniffing between his thighs like a dog. But it turns me right off when he demands it. My arousal drops to zero, *and* I feel annoyed and tense.

And, conversely, just because *you* would ask for something if you really wanted it, don't assume that your partner would too. Women are encouraged to be unselfish in bed to the point of foregoing their own pleasures. She may not *please* you in bed, but it's unlikely to be because she's *selfish*.

In this respect it always pays to take that extra bit of trouble sexually with her. In enjoying your partner's unselfishness you may seem to be doing OK – the 'if she's prepared to do it, why shouldn't I take advantage of it?' sort of attitude. In fact it's quite likely that if you met her halfway *both* your sex lives would be enhanced. You might at least give it a try.

8. *Positions*: one of the most pernicious sex myths is that the more outré the position the 'hotter' the sex will be. Unless your woman is very experienced in orgasm it's unlikely that she will find way-out positions fulfilling. Read the section entitled 'Which Position?' in Chapter 10 and familiarize yourself with some of the advantages and drawbacks that women are conscious of. If you want to help her towards more orgasms, let *her* choose the position. When she is more adept, she'll probably be quite happy to try – and really appreciate – something more adventurous.

9. *Faking*: if you suspect that your partner is faking orgasm, don't get angry. Firstly, you may well be wrong. The way a woman displays her orgasm varies from individual to individual, from day to day, from circumstance to circumstance. Unless you've got a torch and some measuring devices with you there's no way you can tell for certain whether the orgasm is genuine or not.

However hurt and distressed you may feel, you can be quite certain she feels even worse. And if you are right, remember: no woman in the world wants to have to fake, and *of course* we'd all much rather be quite open. Read Chapter 14 and you'll see why we do it none the less. Confronting her will not help either of you, it'll simply make matters more tense. Think of it as a challenge: you will try to work her out of faking naturally. After all, it would be more rewarding if she stopped of her own accord, because sex had become sufficiently arousing to have a genuine orgasm, rather than because you prevented her, making her difficulty public each time you have sex.

Bear in mind the above advice and you'll be well on the way to an improved relationship. Good luck!

BIBLIOGRAPHY

In a few cases I have added a short comment about the book or article which I hope you may find helpful. In most cases I have given the publisher and the edition used, except for those books that are widely available in various editions, in which case I have usually given just the date of the first or most important edition.

Abel, E. L., *Drugs and Sex: A Bibliography*, Greenwood Press, 1983

Allardice, P., *Aphrodisiacs and Love Magic*, Prism Press, 1989

anonymous, *L'Escholle des Filles*. My quote comes from the unattributed translation in Parker's *Anthology of Erotic Prose*.

anonymous, *Les Tableaux Vivants*, English translation, 1888 (quoted in Atkins)

Apollinaire, G., *The Exploits of a Young Don Juan*, A. Lykiard (trans.), Star Books, 1986

Atkins, J., *Sex in Literature*, Vols 1–4, Calder and Boyars, 1970. An invaluable, broad-ranging survey, written with intelligence and humour.

Aubrey, J., *Brief Lives*, O. L. Dick (ed), 1949

Beltrami, E., A. Dupras & R. Tremblay, 'The Effect of Sexual Fantasy Frequencies on the Outcome of Short-term Treatment Program for Sexual Inadequacy in Heterosexual Couples' in *Progress in Sexology*, R. Gemme & C. C. Wheeler (eds), Plenum Press, 1977

Bond, S. B., & D. L. Mosher, 'Guided Imagery of Rape: Fantasy, Reality, and the Willing Victim Myth' in *Journal of Sex Research* Vol. 22, No. 4, May 1986

Boston Women's Health Book Collective, *Our Bodies, Ourselves*, A. Phillips & J. Rakusen (British eds), Penguin Books, 1979. An excellent book: strong, intelligent and informative.

Cleland, J., *Memoirs of a Woman of Pleasure*, 1748–9. Popularly known as *Fanny Hill*.

Cole, M., 'Normal and dysfunctional sexual behaviour: frequencies', in M. Cole & W. Dryden, *Sex Therapy in Britain*, Open University Press, 1988

Crépault, C., G. Abraham, R. Porto & M. Couture, 'Erotic Imagery in Women' in *Progress in Sexology*, R. Gemme & C. C. Wheeler (eds), Plenum Press, 1977

Douglas, N., *The Norman Douglas Limerick Book*, Anthony Blond, 1969

Dworkin, A., *Pornography: Men Possessing Women*, The Women's Press, 1981. Essential reading for anyone interested in the politics of the subject. It's powerful, provocative and bold. For a criticism of Dworkin, try Alison Assiter's *Pornography, Feminism and the Individual*, Pluto Press, 1989

Davidson, J. K., & L. E. Hoffman, 'Sexual Fantasies and Sexual Satisfaction: An Empirical Analysis of Erotic Thought' in *Journal of Sex Research* Vol. 22, No. 2, May 1986

Fisher, Seymour, *The Female Orgasm*, Basic Books, 1973. A huge, relentless survey of all the literature on the subject. Only for the dedicated.

Friday, N., *Men In Love: Their Secret Fantasies*, Arrow, 1980. It was my feeling, after reading this, that they were best kept secret.

Garcia, L. T., et al., 'Sex Difference in Sexual Arousal to Different Erotic Stories' in *Journal of Sex Research* Vol. 20, No. 4, November 1984

Greer, G., *The Change: Women, Aging and the Menopause*, Hamish Hamilton, 1991. Characteristically opinionated; I found it inspiring.

Hello!, 4 January 1992

Harrell, T. H., & R. D. Stolp, 'Effects of Erotic Guided Imagery on Female Sexual Arousal and Emotional Response' in *Journal of Sex Research* Vol. 21, No. 3, August 1985

Harris, F., *My Life and Loves*, Grove Press, 1947

Heiman, J. R., & J. LoPiccolo, *Becoming Orgasmic*, Piatkus, 1988. A competitor! Informative and doubtless well meaning, but its rambling, humourless tone did not inspire me. Why must sex manuals be so *precious*? It is also the source of the ignominious illustration discussed in Chapter 5.

Hemingway, E., *For Whom the Bell Tolls*, Jonathan Cape, 1941

Hite, Shere, *The Hite Report on Female Sexuality*, Pandora, 1989. A fascinating book that I have often referred to.
  The Hite Report on Male Sexuality, Macdonald Optima, 1990. A much longer and less sharp book than the original *Hite Report*, but interesting if you've got the time and stomach for it.

Ibara, S., *Life of an Amorous Woman*, I. Morris (trans.), Chapman and Hall, 1963

Jong, E., *Fear of Flying*, Secker and Warburg, 1974

Kaplan, H. S., *The New Sex Therapy: Active treatment of sexual dysfunction*, Penguin, 1978. Something of a classic.

Kinsey, A. C., W. B. Pomeroy, C. E. Martin & P. H. Gebhard, *Sexual Behaviour in the Human Female*, Saunders, 1953

Kilmartin, A., *Sexual Cystitis*, Arrow Books, 1988. Invaluable even for women who've never had cystitis. I highly recommend all Kilmartin's books.

Kitzinger, S., *Women's Experience of Sex*, Penguin Books, 1985

Krafft-Ebing, R. V., *Psychopathia Sexualis*. First published in 1886, the seventh edition was translated into English in 1892 and continued to influence for a long time. My translation is from the grandly described 'only authorised English adaptation' of the twelfth edition, Physicians and Surgeons Book Company, 1931.

Lazarsfeld, S., *Woman's Experience of the Male*, London, 1940

Leiblum, S. R., & L. A. Pervin, *Principles and Practice of Sex Therapy*, Tavistock Publications, 1980

Lovesey, P., *Rough Cider*, Bodley Head, 1986

Marshall, D. S., & R. C. Suggs (eds), *Human Sexual Behaviour: Variations in the Ethnographic Spectrum*, Spectrum, 1971

Maier, R. A., *Human Sexuality in Perspective*, Nelson Hall, 1984. A good, broad-minded textbook for university students.

Magoun, H. W., 'John B. Watson and the Study of Human Sexual Behaviour' in *Journal of Sex Research* Vol. 17, No. 4, November 1981

Markowitz, H., & W. Brender, 'Patterns of Sexual Responsiveness During the Menstrual Cycle' in *Progress in Sexology*, R. Gemme & C. C. Wheeler (eds), Plenum Press, 1977

Masters, W. H., & V. E. Johnson, *Human Sexual Inadequacy*, Little, Brown and Company, 1970

Masters, W. H., & V. E. Johnson, *Human Sexual Response*, Little, Brown and Company, 1966

McCarthy, M., *The Group*, Weidenfeld and Nicolson, 1963

Moore, G., *Memoirs Of My Dead Life*, London, 1906

Ovid, *The Art of Love*, J. H. Mozley (trans.), Loeb Classical Library, 1929

Percy Folio MS (c. 1620–50). The extract is taken from a verse entitled 'Off a Puritanine', quoted in Atkins.

'Protest by the Medical Profession', quoted in Atkins as being 'after Swinburne'.

Reage, P., *The Story of O*, Corgi, 1972

Reuben, D., *Everything You Always Wanted to Know About Sex . . .*, W. H. Allen, 1970. Whatever it is, you'd be better off asking someone else.

Roding, F., *Some Sort of Spell*, Mills and Boon, 1989

Sparks, J., *The Sexual Connection*, Sphere Books, 1979

Sherfey, M. J., *The Nature and Evolution of Female Sexuality*, Random House, 1972

Stevens, S. D., & A. Klarner, *Deadly Doses: a writer's guide to poisons*, Writer's Digest Books, 1990. A fascinating book, filled with all manner of toxic gruesomeness.

Symons, D., *The Evolution of Human Sexuality*, Oxford University Press, 1979

Sue, David, 'Erotic Fantasies of College Students During Coitus' in *Journal of Sex Research* Vol. 15, No. 4, November 1979

Stimpson, C. R., & E. S. Person, *Women: Sex and Sexuality*, University of Chicago Press, 1980. This collection contains a long list of literary books about sex. Also a whole chapter on women writers.

Taberner, P. V., *Aphrodisiacs – The Science and the Myth*, Croom Helm, 1985

'Teenage Sex' in *Woman's Own*, 25 November 1991

Winn, D., *Below the Belt*, Macdonald Optima, 1987. Very good guide to genito-urinary infections for women. It is direct, clear, informative and with plenty of straightforward advice.

'Woman of the 90s' in *Woman's Own*, 11 November 1991. The quiz itself was entitled 'What Makes You a Woman of the 90s?' in 19 August 1991

Vasyayana, *Kama Sutra*, R. F. Burton & F. F. Arbuthnot (trans.), Unwin Hyman, 1981

Vizinczey, S., *In Praise of Older Women*, Pan, 1967

SUGGESTED READING FOR FANTASY

The trouble with many explicit erotic books is that they are written by men, and often don't ring true on the subject of women and women's desires. Whether or not these limitations bother you you'll have to decide for yourself. I've tried to give a short selection that caters for most literary tastes.

Barbach, L. – has written a number of books about women and sex and edited *Erotic Interludes* and *Pleasures* collections of erotic stories by women. Very American.

Bible. 'The Song of Songs' is a marvellous biblical erotic book. Many consider it the finest in the English language. Some still insist it merely expresses the love between the Church and the Lord, but it's obviously not quite so innocent.

Cavalier Poets – the Earl of Rochester in particular.

Cleland, J., *Memoirs of a Woman of Pleasure*, also known as *Fanny Hill*. The subject of a famous obscenity trial. One of my favourites.

Bibliography

Colette – the *Claudine* stories. Also *Cheri* and *La Fin de Cheri*, about a woman's affair with a younger man.

Defoe, D., *Moll Flanders* and *Roxana*. Stories of mildly libidinous women, but I've always found them pleasantly suggestive.

Friday, N., *My Secret Garden*, Quartet Books, 1979 – a record of women's fantasies. Not all of them the most subtle stuff you'll read, but very encouraging, and her discussions are frank, intelligent and refreshing. If you're interested she's also done a book entitled *Men In Love: their secret fantasies*, Arrow, 1980.

Harris, F., *My Life and Loves*. The greatest of the male self-applaudatory fantasies, but I sometimes find something in it if I'm in the right mood.

Hollander, X., *Emmanuelle* and others in a similar vein.

Jong, E., *Fear of Flying*. Very funny novel about a bored married woman's search for sexual liberation.

Lawrence, D. H., *Lady Chatterley's Lover* – because it's generally considered great literature, people tend to think it full of insight into female sexuality. I've never agreed.

Mills and Boon books I've always had a soft spot for. They're getting more explicit these days, and the sex and courtship can be quite exciting. The heroines nowadays tend to be an odd mixture of fifties housewife and eighties go-getter.

Miller, H., *Tropic of Capricorn*. If you like lots of thrusting and male penile prowess then this is the one for you. Self-indulgent rot if you ask me.

Nin, A., *Little Birds*

Ovid, *Metamorphosis* and *The Art of Love*

Parker, D., *An Anthology of Erotic Prose*, Constable, 1981. Very useful for giving you a wide range of familiar and unfamiliar authors – and giving you an idea of whose books are worth following up.

Vidal, G., *Myra Beckinridge*. A strong, 'significant' book, but I never really felt that I understood the significance, or particularly wanted to.

Vizinczey, S., *In Praise of Older Women*. A sensitive, humorous and very well written book about a young man's exploits after the war.

Zola, E., *Nana*. The story of a French courtesan whose corruption of men's morals is irresistible, and who resorts to women whenever she finds men too unpalatable to endure.

All Pan Books are available at your local bookshop or newsagent, or can be ordered direct from the publisher. Indicate the number of copies required and fill in the form below.

Send to: Macmillan General Books C.S.
             Book Service By Post
             PO Box 29, Douglas I-O-M
             IM99 1BQ

or phone: 01624 675137, quoting title, author and credit card number.

or fax: 01624 670923, quoting title, author, and credit card number.

or Internet: http://www.bookpost.co.uk

Please enclose a remittance* to the value of the cover price plus 75 pence per book for post and packing. Overseas customers please allow £1.00 per copy for post and packing.

*Payment may be made in sterling by UK personal cheque, Eurocheque, postal order, sterling draft or international money order, made payable to Book Service By Post.

Alternatively by Access/Visa/MasterCard

Card No.   ☐☐☐☐☐☐☐☐☐☐☐☐☐☐☐☐

Expiry Date   ☐☐☐☐☐☐☐☐☐☐☐☐☐☐☐☐

Signature   _____

Applicable only in the UK and BFPO addresses.

While every effort is made to keep prices low, it is sometimes necessary to increase prices at short notice. Pan Books reserve the right to show on covers and charge new retail prices which may differ from those advertised in the text or elsewhere.

NAME AND ADDRESS IN BLOCK CAPITAL LETTERS PLEASE

Name _____

Address _____

_____

_____

_____

8/95

Please allow 28 days for delivery.
Please tick box if you do not wish to receive any additional information. ☐